Influenza

Jan Wilschut PhD
Professor of Molecular Virology
Department of Medical Microbiology,
University of Groningen,
Groningen, the Netherlands

Janet E McElhaney MD
Associate Professor
Center for Immunotherapy of Cancer and
Infectious Diseases,
University of Connecticut Health Center,
Farmington, Connecticut, USA

Mosby

MOSBY
An imprint of Elsevier Limited.

The
Publisher's
policy is to use
**paper manufactured
from sustainable forests**

ISBN 07234 33852

Cataloguing in Publication Data
Catalogue records for this book are available from the US Library of Congress and the British Library.

Note
Medical knowledge is constantly changing. As new information becomes available, changes in treatment, procedures, equipment and the use of drugs become necessary. The editors/authors/contributors and the publishers have taken care to ensure that the information given in this text is accurate and up to date. However, readers are strongly advised to confirm that the information, especially with regard to drug usage, complies with the latest legislation and standards of practice.

Printed by Grafos, Spain.

Acknowledgements

During the course of this project, we have been priviliged to work with the editorial team of *Infectious Diseases*, 2nd Edition (Mosby), and we would like to thank team-members Jonathan Cohen, Timothy Kiehn, William Powderly and Jan Verhoef for their thorough review of this book.

We would also like to thank Bram Palache from Solvay Pharmaceuticals (Weesp, The Netherlands) for his critical evaluation of the manuscript. Bram has been very supportive and his valuable suggestions and comments have contributed greatly to the final result. In addition, in the early and late stages of this project, respectively, Maurice Gleeson and James Ryan made important contributions to the manuscript.

We have highly appreciated the cooperation with the Elsevier project team, and we would like to thank in particular project manager Elisabeth Lawrence and editorial manager Alison Taylor for their efforts in bringing this – sometimes challenging – project to a proper end on time.

Finally, we wish to thank those who provided us with figures, references or suggestions, including René Benne, Walter Beyer, Robert Bittman, Laura Bungener, André van Eerde, Ted van Essen, Ron Fouchier, Lysia Gerez, Anke Huckriede, Jeroen Medema, and Guus Rimmelzwaan...

... and we thank our colleagues in the lab and families at home for their patience.

Jan Wilschut
Janet McElhaney
Groningen and Farmington, August 2004

Foreword

Last century, three major influenza pandemics have been responsible for at least 50 million deaths worldwide. In addition, annual influenza winter epidemics have an enormous medical and economic impact on society. It is widely documented that serious morbidity and mortality occur among the elderly. Also, influenza frequently leads to complications in young children. Yet despite this, many people, including health care professionals, underestimate the importance of the disease.

As stated by the World Health Organization, annual influenza vaccination is the cornerstone for prevention and control. Efficacious influenza vaccines have been available for over 50 years. Nevertheless, their potential to control influenza is not fully exploited. In light of the recent avian influenza virus outbreaks and associated concerns about a new influenza pandemic, many public health authorities stress the need to expand efforts to minimize the annual burden of influenza and to improve pandemic preparedness.

This book provides an overview of influenza, its pathogenesis, epidemiology, the burden of disease and its health economics. It also summarizes available information on the molecular biology of influenza and the emergence of new influenza viruses. It is written primarily for health care professionals, so they may understand the facts behind increased efforts to implement immunization policies recommended by health authorities in many countries.

The book recognizes the key role of general practitioners in the prevention and treatment of influenza for the benefit of their patients and society. By publishing this book, the authors contribute to international efforts to emphasize the major burden of influenza and the need for better control.

Albert D.M.E Osterhaus
Professor of Virology
Erasmus MC, Rotterdam, the Netherlands

Contents

Abbreviations

ADCC	antibody-dependent cell-mediated cytotoxicity
APC	antigen-presenting cell
ca	cold-adapted
CHF	congestive heart failure
CT	cholera toxin
CTAB	cetyl trimethyl ammonium bromide
CTL	cytotoxic T lymphocyte
DC	dendritic cell
ER	endoplasmic reticulum
GBS	Guillain–Barré syndrome
GM-CSF	granulocyte–macrophage colony-stimulating factor
Grz B	granzyme B
HA	haemagglutinin
HI	haemagglutination–inhibition
ICER	incremental cost-effectiveness ratio
IFN	interferon
IL	interleukin
ILI	influenza-like illness
ISCOM	immune-stimulating complex
LAIV	live attenuated influenza vaccine
LT	*E. coli* heat-labile enterotoxin
LTB	recombinant B subunit of *E. coli* heat-labile enterotoxin
MHC	major histocompatibility complex
MRP	Mutual Recognition Procedure
NA	neuraminidase
NK	natural killer (cells)
NP	nucleoprotein
PCR	polymerase chain reaction
RMS	Reference Member State
RNP	ribonucleoprotein

RSV	respiratory syncytial virus
sIgA	secretory immunoglobulin A
SRD	single radial immunodiffusion
SRH	single radial haemolysis
TGN	trans-Golgi network
Th	T helper (cell)
TLR	toll-like receptor
TNF	tumour necrosis factor
URI	upper respiratory illness
URTI	upper respiratory tract infection

Introduction

The highly contagious, acute, febrile, respiratory illness, referred to as "influenza" or simply "flu", has been known for centuries. It occurs in epidemics of variable severity almost every winter and in occasional major pandemic outbreaks.[1–3] The term "influenza" was derived from the Italian *influentia* in the mid-1300s, indicating that the illness was believed to result from astrological influences. Yet, at the time, the aetiology of the disease and the explanation for its peculiar behaviour remained elusive. At the turn of the 19th century, influenza was thought to be due to a bacterial infection with *Haemophilus influenzae*. It was not until 1931 that Richard Shope[4] showed that swine influenza could be transmitted with filtered mucus, indicating that the causative agent was probably a virus. A few years later, Smith and co-workers[5] isolated the influenza virus from humans with respiratory illness.

Even today, "flu" is a major, and often underestimated, burden for society, from both clinical and economic points of view.[6] This relates not only to the occasional major pandemic outbreaks of influenza, but also to the recurring annual winter epidemics. Fortunately, since the virus was first discovered, efficient means to contain the infection have been developed. Vaccination is the cornerstone of influenza prevention and control (see pp. 124–151). Accordingly, the World Health Organization (WHO) has issued guidelines for the implementation of influenza vaccination programmes in individual countries.[7,8] As a result, many thousands of lives are saved worldwide each year. Yet, in many places, implementation of vaccination programmes is woefully deficient.[9] This implies that significant numbers of people at risk for the complications of influenza remain vulnerable to infection and possibly death. The primary-care physician is in a key position to address difficulties with implementing these public health policies in his or her own practice.

Key Messages

- The impact of influenza is often underestimated – annual epidemics are deadly and costly events, and pandemic outbreaks may be devastating.
- Deaths can be prevented and cost savings made by appropriate vaccination practice.
- Many people who need vaccination do not get it.
- Primary-care physicians play a pivotal role in reducing morbidity and mortality from influenza by vaccinating people at risk for its complications.

The influenza virus

Influenza virions are enveloped particles of spherical or elongated shape, measuring 80–120 nm in diameter and containing a segmented, single-stranded, negative-sense RNA genome (see pp. 23–44).[10,11] The influenza virus belongs to the family Orthomyxoviridae. There are three influenza virus genera, or antigenic types, within this family: influenza A, B and C. The influenza A viruses have been responsible for the major pandemics of influenza in the last century and are also the causative agents for most of the annual outbreaks of epidemic influenza. Therefore, this book will be limited mostly to a discussion of the characteristics and impact of influenza A viruses.

Figure 1 presents an electron micrograph of the influenza A virus. A characteristic feature of the virus is its outermost layer of spike-like projections. These are the two viral surface glycoproteins, haemagglutinin (HA) and neuraminidase (NA), which are embedded in the lipid membrane of the viral envelope. HA, the major spike protein, is responsible for attachment of the virus to specific receptors on the host cell surface. HA also mediates a fusion reaction between the viral envelope and the cell membrane,

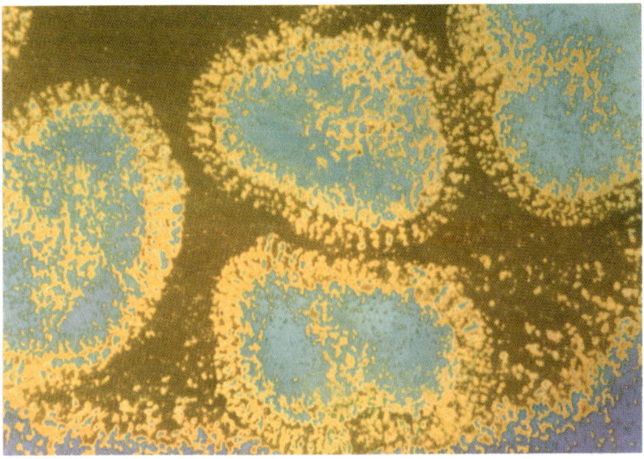

Figure 1. Influenza virus. Copyright © Ron Boardman; Frank Lane Picture Agency/CORBIS.

through which the viral genome gains access to the interior of the cell (see pp. 23–44). Once inside the cell, the viral RNA is replicated and viral proteins are synthesized, leading to the production of many thousands of new virus particles per cell. Ultimately, the cell dies as a result of the infection. In the lungs and airways, this process of cell lysis leads to desquamation of the respiratory epithelium as one aspect of influenza pathogenesis.

Antigenic variability of influenza: origin of pandemics and epidemics

There are many different influenza A virus subtypes, depending on the nature of the HA and NA glycoproteins on their surface.[10,11] Fifteen different HA and nine different NA subtypes have been identified. These subtypes are distinguishable serologically, which means that antibodies to one subtype do not react with another subtype. All HA and NA subtypes circulate in aquatic birds. Only some of these subtypes (H1, H2 and H3; N1 and N2) have been identified in human influenza viruses.

Influenza pandemics are the result of so-called antigenic

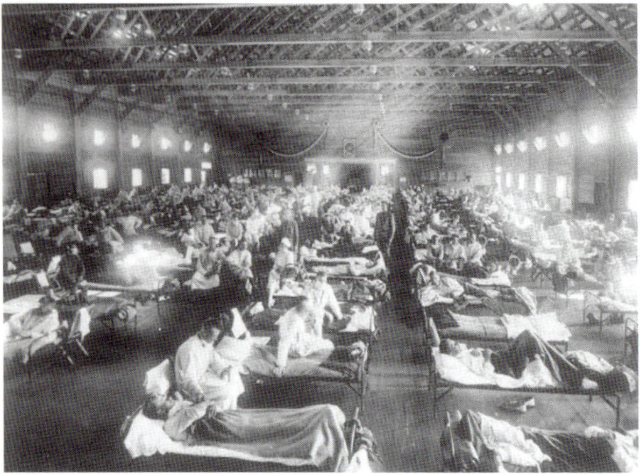

Figure 2. Emergency hospital during the influenza epidemic 1918, Camp Funston, Kansas. Courtesy of the National Museum of Health and Medicine, Armed Forces Institute of Pathology, Washington, D.C. (NCP1603).

shift of the virus (see pp. 45–67).[11] This means that a virus with a new HA (and NA) subtype is introduced into humans. Since the population is immunologically naive to that new virus subtype, the infection may spread rapidly and cause high morbidity and mortality among the entire population, including young healthy people.[2] Three major influenza pandemics spread around the globe in the 20th century. The Spanish flu (caused by an H1N1 influenza A virus) struck in 1918–19, after the First World War, and resulted in the deaths of at least 40 million people, more than the war itself (Figure 2). Other pandemics occurred in 1957 (Asian flu, H2N2) and 1968 (Hong Kong flu, H3N2). Antigenic shifts appear to occur as a result of so-called genetic reassortment within cells dually infected with two different influenza viruses (see pp. 45–67).[12]

The current information supports the concept that reassorted influenza viruses are derived from avian influenza reservoirs.[11,13–15] Avian influenza can be transmitted to humans, with pigs possibly acting as an intermediary host in which reassortment takes place. Highly pathogenic avian influenza virus may also be directly transmitted to humans, as became evident for the first time during the H5N1 chicken flu ("fowl plague") outbreak in Hong Kong in 1997. In this incident, 18 people were infected with the avian virus, six of whom died.[16] Similarly, in 2003, an outbreak of fowl plague (H7N7 subtype) in the Netherlands resulted in the direct transmission of the virus to poultry workers and veterinarians, killing one person.[17] Furthermore, in 2004, an outbreak of highly pathogenic H5N1 chicken flu in South-East Asia resulted in a number of human infections in Vietnam and Thailand, with a very high case-fatality rate, underscoring the disconcerting reality of an influenza pandemic threat.

In addition to genetic reassortment resulting in the formation of new human influenza virus subtypes, established virus subtypes undergo significant antigenic adaptation, referred to as antigenic drift (see pp. 45–67).[11] Antigenic drift involves minor changes in the HA and NA that occur as a result of mutations in the viral genome, resulting in amino acid substitutions in antigenic sites. These changes may render the new strain different enough to at least partially avoid the immunity induced by previous strains. Thus, new influenza epidemics may arise. In the temperate regions, these epidemics generally occur in the winter months (from October to March in the northern hemisphere, and from April to September in the southern hemisphere).

Clinical picture and impact of flu

Transmission and pathogenesis

After being inhaled by droplet transmission, the influenza virus attacks the respiratory epithelium and commandeers the host cell's replication machinery to produce new progeny virus particles, which further infect other cells (see pp. 23–44 and pp. 86–106). "Innate" immune responses retard the initial spread of the virus in the respiratory tract and provide valuable time for the host to mount a specific "adaptive" immune response against the invading virus. B-lymphocytes produce antibodies that bind to and neutralize the virus on the mucosal surfaces, while T-lymphocytes dispose of the infected cells that have become factories for producing new virus particles (see pp. 68–85).

The body's immune response to influenza (see pp. 68–85) produces a number of inflammatory cytokines, which are responsible for most of the symptoms of influenza. Except in rare circumstances, the virus remains limited to the respiratory epithelium (see pp. 23–44). Thus, the major systemic symptoms such as fever, myalgia and malaise are caused by these circulating cytokines. Influenza is generally a self-limited disease. However, in the complete absence of immunity to a specific subtype of influenza, such as with the emergence of a novel pandemic strain, even young people may die within 24–48 hours of the onset of symptoms, the overwhelming inflammatory response to the virus causing an acute respiratory distress-like syndrome. Inadequate immune responses as often occur in the very young and very old may lead to a primary viral pneumonia or secondary bacterial infection (see pp. 86–106).

Impact of influenza epidemics and pandemics

Influenza epidemics have been recognized as a major cause of morbidity and increased mortality, especially in the very young, the very old, people with chronic cardiopulmonary conditions, pregnant women and immunocompromised individuals (see pp. 107–123). Each year, influenza results in 3–5 million cases of severe illness and kills between 0.25 and 0.5 million people worldwide.[6,18] The WHO estimates that there are currently 1000 million people worldwide who are at high risk of suffering or dying from influenza and its complications.[18]

As the elderly population increases, future influenza epidemics will be associated with ever-increasing hospitalization rates and excess mortality unless adequate prophylactic measures are taken. In developed countries, about 100 people per million population die annually from influenza.[6,19] Most of these deaths (95%) occur in those over 60 years of age (12%, 29% and 54% in people aged 60–69, 70–79 and >80 years respectively).[20]

Even though the three major pandemic outbreaks of influenza in the 20th century have caused many millions of deaths, it has been estimated that the cumulative mortality of annual influenza epidemics in the last century exceeded that of the three major pandemic outbreaks.[6,21] This underscores the fact that not only influenza pandemics but also the recurrent annual outbreaks of flu remain a major health threat worldwide. Thus, public health policy needs to address the interrelated issues of optimizing both the effectiveness of annual vaccination programmes and the preparedness for future pandemic outbreaks of influenza. Primary-care physicians play a key role in this regard by participating in influenza surveillance and by providing appropriate preventive and treatment regimens for their patients.

Prevention and control

Vaccination

Vaccination remains the cornerstone of influenza prevention (see pp. 124–151). Inactivated influenza vaccines have been in use for the past 60 years (Figure 3). These vaccines have an excellent safety and efficacy record.

The WHO recommends annual vaccination of people in at-risk groups.[7,8] The primary target groups for annual

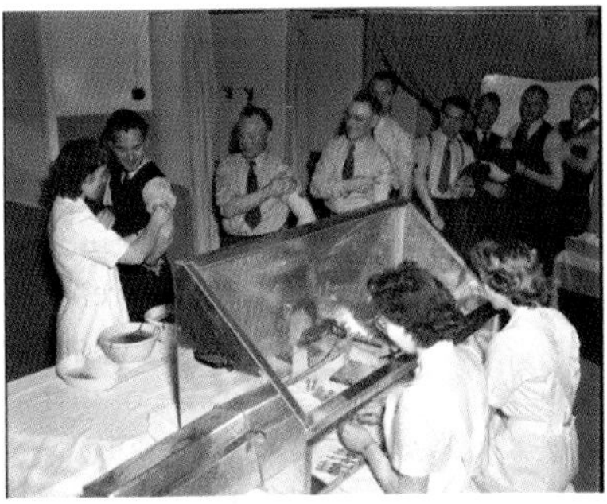

Figure 3. Influenza vaccination in 1950s. Photo courtesy of Solvay Pharmaceuticals, Weesp, the Netherlands.

vaccination include the elderly, nursing home residents, patients with chronic respiratory or cardiovascular disease, diabetes or renal dysfunction, as well as immunocompromised individuals. In addition, it is also recommended that health care workers and family members of people in high-risk groups be vaccinated.

The clinical effectiveness and cost-effectiveness of inactivated influenza vaccines have been clearly demonstrated.[22] For example, vaccination of community-dwelling senior citizens reduces hospitalization rates for pneumonia or other respiratory conditions by >30% and death from all causes by 50%. For nursing home residents the benefits of influenza vaccination are even more striking, with reductions of hospitalization rates or death from all causes of 48% and 68%, respectively (see pp. 124–151).

However, despite the established effectiveness of immunization, the national and international response to influenza prevention is often inadequate (see pp. 124–151). In many countries, the established benefits of vaccination have not been translated into effective immunization programmes. Only 50 countries have policies for influenza immunization and only 10–20% of people in high-risk groups are protected.[9,18] While we do have the means to prevent the serious consequences of influenza, the implementation of preventive measures remains suboptimal, and as a consequence, currently, the majority

> "The relatively low uptake of influenza vaccines in most industrialized countries implies that significant proportions of the groups at risk of complications from influenza are not vaccinated. WHO strongly emphasizes the importance of raising the public consciousness of influenza and its complications as well as of the beneficial effects of influenza vaccination."
>
> ***World Health Organization*** **(Ref. 8; Appendix 2)**

of at-risk individuals is unprotected and vulnerable to infection and death.

Antivirals

While vaccination is the method of choice for influenza prophylaxis, under specific conditions where the individual has not been or cannot be vaccinated, or is not fully protected by vaccination, the use of antiviral drugs should be considered for treatment or prevention of influenza infection (see pp. 152–165). In this regard, the primary-care physician needs to know whether influenza is circulating in the community and how to diagnose influenza illness for the purpose of appropriate prescription of influenza antiviral drugs.

Antiviral drugs approved for treament or prophylaxis of influenza include the M2 channel inhibitors amantidine and rimantidine, and the neuraminidase inhibitors zanamivir and oseltamivir. The application of these drugs to clinical practice may be limited by issues of efficacy with respect to the type of influenza virus (influenza A vs. B), drug resistance, adverse effects and cost. In the case of the M2 ion channel blockers, these drugs are only effective against influenza A, the induction of drug resistance is well documented and side-effects can be significant, especially in older people. While these issues have not been apparent with the more recent neuraminidase inhibitors, their cost may be prohibitive for broad use of these medications, and for the inhaled zanamivir there is a caution against its use in cases of airway hypersensitivity. These issues not only limit the use of antivirals for individual treatment, but also present some major challenges to their use in potential future pandemics.

Pandemic preparedness

Since the 1997 H5N1 avian flu outbreak in Hong Kong, the need for intensified efforts to control the potential pandemic threat of influenza has been widely recognized. This is reflected by a resolution of the World Health

Assembly urging member states to increase their efforts toward influenza prevention.[18] It is only a matter of time before another pandemic influenza virus emerges. This will inevitably result in a new global outbreak with the deaths of millions of people unless preventive measures are adequately instituted. However, there is a serious lack of national and global preparedness for a future influenza pandemic. Just a few countries, including Canada (see Appendix 1), have formal, legally sanctioned, pandemic preparedness plans. Co-ordination of pandemic preparedness at the global level is hindered by the lack of such national plans, and by inadequate information on the projected need for vaccine doses, antiviral drugs and associated supplies. In the current situation, no country will have vaccines at the start of the next pandemic and it will take at least 6 months after the first detection of the new pandemic virus before significant quantities of vaccine will become available. Thus, despite the fact that experts and the WHO are expecting a new pandemic to occur, individual countries and the world are not sufficiently prepared to contain such a potential global health threat. A potentially disastrous pandemic was averted in 1997 and 2004 by mass culling of poultry during the outbreaks of avian influenza in South-East Asia (Figure 4). The fear was that this highly pathogenic virus, with a very high mortality rate among infected humans, would adapt within its human host and develop enhanced transmissibility from human to human. Although, fortunately, this fear did not materialize at the time, the risk remains. Strategies that decrease morbidity and mortality and improve the effectiveness of vaccination against annual epidemics will contribute to future planning for the next pandemic. According to the WHO, one way to increase pandemic preparedness is to increase interpandemic vaccine supply. This would enlarge vaccine production capacity, which will subsequently increase vaccine availability in the case of a pandemic. At the same time, increased vaccine use during

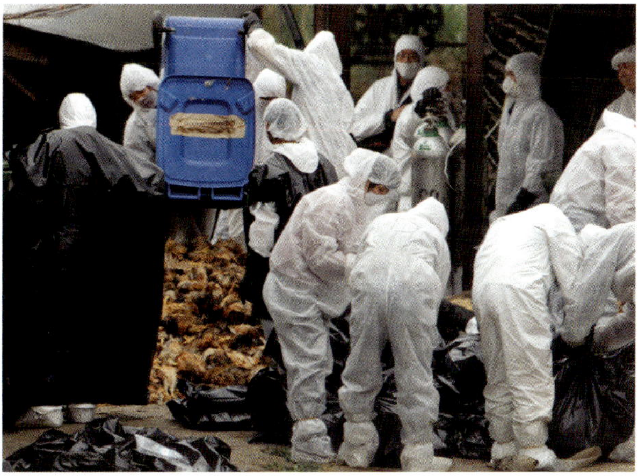

Figure 4. Culling of chickens at a Hong Kong farm following an outbreak of avian flu. Copyright © Reuters/CORBIS.

interpandemic periods will reduce the annual burden of the disease.[18]

Role of the primary-care physician

As indicated above, the WHO recommends annual immunization of at-risk individuals as the best and most cost-effective strategy for reducing influenza-related morbidity and mortality.[7,8,18] However, there is often a gap between what policy-makers want and what actually happens in practice, because the links between policy-makers and primary-care physicians are generally loose. Policy-makers cannot take into account all the logistical difficulties that the primary-care physician faces, and policy needs to be translated into guidelines and recommendations specific for each local area.

Primary-care physicians are in an optimal position to promote preventive measures for both epidemic and pandemic influenza containment. On the basis of the available evidence, offering vaccination to at-risk patients should be considered an ethical obligation.[23] By ensuring that all people in target groups are vaccinated, the primary-care physician can make a significant contribution to public health. There are many factors that hinder the effective vaccination of people at high risk (reimbursement, public awareness, vaccine supply), but one factor that this book hopes to address is the lack of guidance for health care professionals involved in implementing vaccination policies. Ultimately, if primary-care physicians reading this book were to vaccinate the majority of their at-risk patients, this activity would go a long way toward ameliorating the burden of future influenza epidemics and pandemics.

The WHO also emphasizes the frequently low level of vaccination of health care personnel working in direct contact with the elderly at-risk group. This is of particular concern because of the strong evidence that health care staff inadvertently assist in the spread of influenza in institutions caring for the elderly, because of the vulnerability of the health care system when staff are ill, and because of the personal well-being of the health care staff involved. The WHO encourages initiatives to raise awareness of influenza and influenza immunization among health care workers.[8] This book is such an initiative.

References

1. Patterson KD. Pandemic and epidemic influenza, 1830–1848. *Soc Sci Med* 1985; **21**: 571–580.

2. Ghendon Y. Introduction to pandemic influenza through history. *Eur J Epidemiol* 1994; **10**: 451–453.

3. Beveridge WI. The chronicle of influenza epidemics. *Hist Phil Life Sci* 1991; **13**: 223–234.

4. Shope RE. Swine influenza. III. Filtration experiments and etiology. *J Exp Med* 1931; **54**: 373–380.

5. Smith W, Andrewes C, Laidlaw P. A virus obtained from influenza patients. *Lancet* 1933; **2**: 66–68.

6. Nicholson KG, Wood JM, Zambon M. Influenza. *Lancet* 2003; **362**: 1733–1745.

7. World Health Organization. Influenza vaccines. *Wkly Epidemiol Rec* 2000; **75**: 281–288.

8. World Health Organization. Influenza vaccines. *Wkly Epidemiol Rec* 2002; **77**: 230–239.

9. Van Essen GA, Forleo E, Palache AM, Fedson DS. Influenza vaccination in 2000: vaccination recommendations and vaccine use in 50 developed and developing countries. *Vaccine* 2003; **21**: 1780–1785.

10. Lamb RA, Krug RM. Orthomyxoviridae: the viruses and their replication. In: Knipe DM, Howley PM, Griffin DE *et al*., editors. Fields *Virology*, 4th edn. Lippincott Williams & Wilkins, 2001; pp. 1487–1531.

11. Wright PF, Webster RG. Orthomyxoviruses. In: Knipe DM, Howley PM, Griffin DE *et al*., editors. Fields *Virology*, 4th edn. Lippincott Williams & Wilkins, 2001; pp. 1533–1579.

12. Ito T, Couceiro JN, Kelm S *et al*. Molecular basis for the generation in pigs of influenza A viruses with pandemic potential. *J Virol* 1998; **72**: 7367–7373.

13. Subbarao K, Katz J. Avian influenza viruses infecting humans. *Cell Molec Life Sci* 2000; **57**: 1770–1784.

14. Webster RG. Influenza virus: transmission between species and relevance to emergence of the next human pandemic. *Arch Virol Suppl* 1997; **13**: 105–113.

15. Zambon M. The pathogenesis of influenza in humans. *Rev Med Virol* 2001; **11**(4): 227–241.

16. Claas EC, Osterhaus AD *et al*. Human influenza A H5N1 virus related to a highly pathogenic avian influenza virus. *Lancet* 1998; **351**: 472–477.

17. Fouchier RAM, Schneeberger PM, Rozendaal FW *et al*. Avian influenza A virus (H7N7) associated with human conjunctivitis and a fatal case of acute respiratory distress syndrome. *Proc Natl Acad Sci USA* 2004; **101**: 1356–1361.

18. Influenza: Report by the WHO Secretariat for 111th Session of the WHO Executive Board, January 2003.

Document EB111/10, WHO, November 2002. www.who.int/gb/EB_WHA/PDF/EB111/eeb11110.pdf

19. Barker WH, Mullooly JP. Impact of epidemic type A influenza in a defined adult population. *Am J Epidemiol* 1980; **112**: 798–811.

20. Sprenger MJ, Mulder PG, Beyer WE *et al*. Impact of influenza on mortality in relation to age and underlying disease, 1967–1989. *Int J Epidemiol* 1993; **22**: 334–340.

21. Simonson L, Clarke MJ, Williamson GD *et al*. The impact of influenza epidemics on mortality: introducing a severity index. *Am J Public Health* 1997; **87**: 1944–1950.

22. Nichol KL. The efficacy, effectiveness and cost-effectiveness of inactivated influenza virus vaccines. *Vaccine* 2003; **21**: 1769–1775.

23. Palache A. Influenza vaccines. A reappraisal of their use. *Drugs* 1997; **54**: 841–856.

The Influenza Virus: Structure and Replication

Influenza viruses are enveloped RNA viruses, belonging to the family Orthomyxoviridae.[1] There are three influenza virus genera within this family, influenza A, B and C, distinguishable on the basis of antigenic differences between their matrix and nucleoproteins (M and NP). Influenza A, B and C viruses also differ with respect to host range, variability of the surface glycoproteins, genome organization and morphology.[1] The influenza A viruses are responsible for major pandemic outbreaks of influenza and for most of the well-known annual flu epidemics.[2] Therefore, the discussion here will be limited primarily to influenza A viruses, only referring to influenza B where appropriate. Influenza C virus, which is substantially different from the A and B viruses, is of little importance for human influenza infections, causing only a mild common-cold-like disease; it will not be further discussed in this book.

The A and B viruses contain two major envelope glycoproteins, haemagglutinin (HA) and neuraminidase (NA).[1] An important feature of influenza viruses is their segmented genome, the A and B viruses containing eight independent RNA segments of negative polarity. The RNA segments are packaged in the viral core. The core is surrounded by a lipid membrane, or "envelope", derived from the plasma membrane of the infected host cell during the process of budding of progeny virus from the cell's surface.[1]

After transmission of influenza virus through aerosols, spread into the environment by a sneezing or coughing infected individual,[3] the virus attacks primarily epithelial cells of the upper and lower respiratory tract.[2] Infection occurs by binding of the viral HA to sialic acid-containing receptors on the target cell surface and subsequent fusion of the viral envelope with the host cell membrane.[1] It is through this fusion process that the viral RNA gains access to the cytosol of the host cell. The RNA then enters the nucleus of the cell, where it is replicated. Viral proteins are being synthesized in the cytosol, ultimately resulting in production of many new virus particles. During the production of progeny virus, the host cell's own protein synthesis is effectively shut down. Finally, having produced many thousands of new virus particles, the cell lyses and dies as a result of the infection.[1]

Key Messages

- There are three types of influenza virus: A, B and C. Influenza A viruses are responsible for all pandemic and most epidemic outbreaks, influenza B viruses also cause human disease, but influenza C virus is of little clinical importance.
- Influenza A and B viruses have two major envelope glycoproteins, haemagglutinin (HA) and neuraminidase (NA). HA is responsible for infectious entry of the virus into cells; it is also the virus' most important surface antigen, against which virus-neutralizing antibodies are directed.
- Influenza virus enters cells through receptor-mediated endocytosis and low-pH-induced fusion from within acidic endosomes.
- Cleavage into two subunits is essential for HA to mediate entry of influenza virus into cells. The HA1 subunit is involved in receptor binding, HA2 has membrane fusion activity.
- The receptor for HA is sialic acid bound to glycolipids or glycoproteins on the host cell surface. Avian and human influenza A viruses have a different receptor specificity; pigs have receptors for both avian and human viruses.
- NA cleaves the sialic acid receptor, thus releasing progeny virus from the infected cell surface. It is the target for the antiviral drugs zanamivir and oseltamivir, which are sialic acid analogues and inhibit progeny virus release.
- Influenza viruses have a segmented RNA genome of negative polarity. Mixed infection of a single cell with two different influenza viruses may lead to genetic reassortment between the two viruses.

Classification and nomenclature of influenza viruses

Influenza A viruses are divided into subtypes, based on the nature of their surface glycoproteins, HA and NA.[1] There are 15 HA and nine NA subtypes, which are distinguishable serologically, i.e. antibodies to one subtype do not react with another. All HA and NA subtypes circulate in aquatic birds.[4] Only some of these subtypes have been identified in influenza viruses isolated from humans or other mammals (Table 1). For humans, influenza virus subtypes include H1N1, H2N2 and H3N2 viruses, corresponding to the three major pandemics of the last century. During recent outbreaks of highly pathogenic avian influenza, there have been rare transmissions of H5N1, H7N7 and H9N2 viruses to humans. Besides humans, influenza A viruses are known to also infect a variety of other mammals, including pigs, horses, seals, whales, mink and non-human primates, as well as birds, serving as a reservoir for influenza A viruses.[1,2,4] There are no influenza B virus subtypes. The B virus primarily infects humans, although recently it has also been isolated from seals.[5]

The current nomenclature system for influenza A viruses includes the host of origin, geographic location of first isolation, strain number and year of isolation.[6] The HA and NA subtype of influenza A viruses is specified in parentheses, e.g. A/Swine/lowa/15/30 (H1N1). By convention, the host of origin of human strains is omitted, e.g. A/Puerto Rico/8/34 (H1N1). Since there are no subtypes of influenza B virus, no parenthetical specification is given in this case and, as the B viruses primarily infect humans, the host of origin is not mentioned in the influenza B virus nomenclature, e.g. B/Yamagata/16/88.

Influenza virus structure

Influenza viruses are roughly spherical, although somewhat pleomorphic, particles, ranging from 80 to 120 nm in diameter.[1,7] Figure 5 presents a model of the overall structure of the influenza virus. A characteristic feature of

Natural hosts of influenza A viruses			
Haemagglutinin		**Neuraminidase**	
Designation	**Predominant hosts**	**Designation**	**Predominant hosts**
H1	Human, pig, birds	N1	Human, pig, birds
H2	Human, pig, birds	N2	Human, pig, birds
H3	Birds, human, pig, horse	N3	Birds
H4	Birds	N4	Birds
H5	Birds, (human)	N5	Birds
H6	Birds	N6	Birds
H7	Birds, horse, (human)	N7	Horse, birds
H8	Birds	N8	Horse, birds
H9	Birds, (human)	N9	Birds
H10	Birds		
H11	Birds		
H12	Birds		
H13	Birds		
H14	Birds		
H15	Birds		

Table 1. Natural hosts of influenza A viruses. The table indicates the subtypes of haemagglutinin (HA) and neuraminidase (NA), and the hosts in which they have been identified. Adapted from Lamb RA, Krug RM. *Orthomyxoviridae*: the viruses and their replication. In: Knipe DM, Howley PM, Griffin DE *et al.*, editors. Fields *Virology*, 4th edn. Lippincott Williams & Wilkins, 2001; pp. 1487–1531[1] with permission from Lippincott Williams & Wilkins.

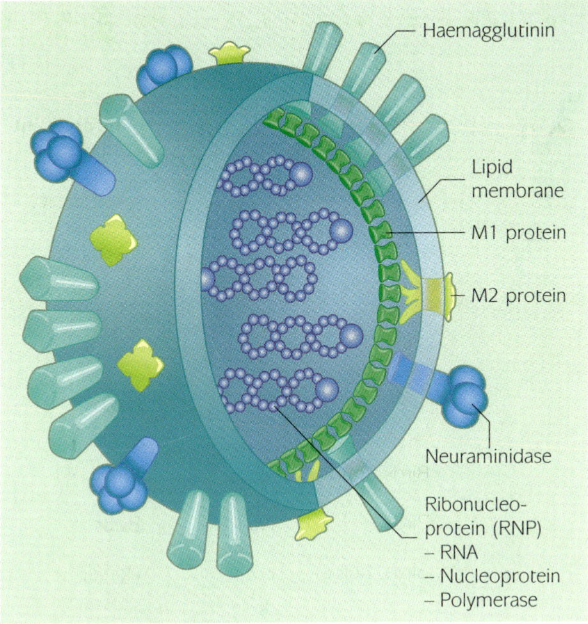

Figure 5. Model of influenza virus.

influenza virus particles is their external layer of approximately 500 spike-like projections. These spikes represent the HA (which has a rod-like shape) and NA (which is mushroom-shaped) glycoproteins.[7] The HA spike is a trimer, consisting of three individual HA monomers,[8] while the NA spike is a tetramer.[9,10] HA is about four times more abundant than NA.

The viral envelope proteins

The major envelope glycoprotein HA is synthesized in the infected cell as an approximately 560 amino acid residue long single polypeptide chain (HA0), which is subsequently cleaved into two subunits, HA1 and HA2.[1,8] These subunits remain covalently linked to one another through disulphide bonds. Cleavage of HA0 is essential for the molecule to be able to mediate membrane fusion between the viral envelope and the host cell membrane, as discussed in more detail below. HA is one of the first proteins for which the entire three-dimensional structure has been elucidated. Treatment of whole virions with the enzyme bromelain, which clips the polypeptide chain just above the viral

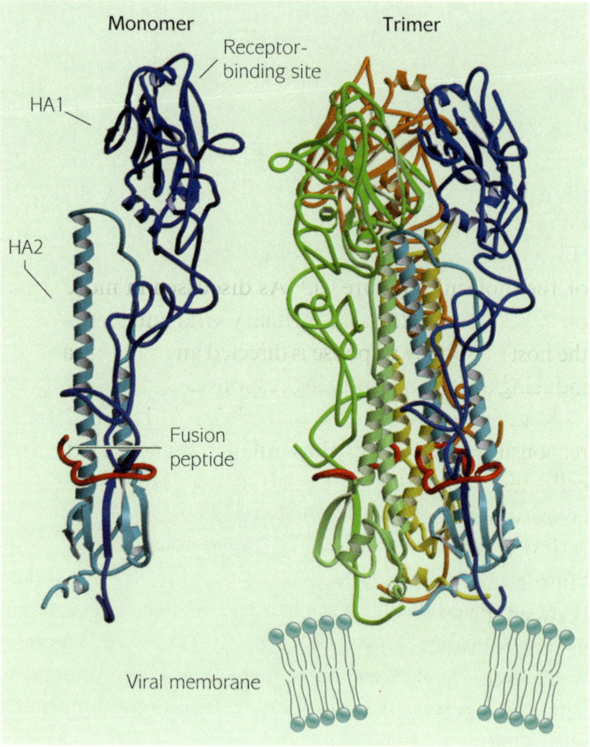

Figure 6. The three-dimensional structure of the influenza haemagglutinin (HA). The HA monomer (left) and trimer (right) are shown. In the monomer, the globular HA1 subunit is shown in dark blue, the HA2 subunit in light blue, with the "fusion peptide" in red. The receptor-binding site of HA1 is located at the tip of the molecule. This figure was produced by André van Eerde (University of Groningen), using MOLSCRIPT, on the basis of the coordinate file from the Protein Data Bank, code 3HMG. Weis WI *et al*. Refinement of the influenza virus hemagglutinin by simulated annealing. *J Molec Biol* 1990; **212**: 737–761.

membrane, releases a water-soluble fragment of the HA spike, commonly referred to as BHA. The ectodomain of HA of A/Aichi/2/68 (H3N2) virus, related to the Hong Kong pandemic virus of 1968, has thus been crystallized and subjected to X-ray analysis.[8,11] Figure 6 presents a representation of the 3D structure of HA based on this pioneering X-ray crystallographic structure determination.

The HA spike protrudes approximately 13.5 nm from the viral surface.[11,12] HA1 and HA2 appear in the structure of the spike as distinct subunits. HA1, the globular domain at the distal end of the spike, is responsible for binding of the virus to its cellular sialic acid receptor, the receptor-binding pocket being located at the very tip of the molecule (Figure 6).[12] HA1 also contains the major antigenic epitopes of the molecule (Figure 7).[13] As discussed in more detail on pages 68–85, HA is the primary viral antigen to which the host's antibody response is directed and the only antigen inducing a virus-neutralizing response.

HA2 forms the fibrous stem of the viral spike. HA2 is responsible for fusion of the viral membrane with the host cell membrane. The N-terminus of HA2 contains a conserved stretch of 20, mostly hydrophobic, amino acid residues. This sequence is generally referred to as the "fusion peptide"; it triggers the membrane fusion process between the viral envelope and the host cell membrane,[11,12] as mentioned above and discussed in more detail below.

The second envelope glycoprotein NA has enzymatic activity, cleaving sialic acid residues from glycoproteins or glycolipids.[9] Since sialic acid-containing glycoproteins or glycolipids function as cellular receptors for attachment of influenza virions, the neuraminidase activity of NA, cleaving such receptors,[14] mediates the release of newly formed virus particles from the surface of infected cells.[15] NA is the target for the antiviral drugs oseltamivir (Tamiflu®) and zanamivir (Relenza®) (see pp. 152–165). These drugs are sialic acid analogues,[16] which inhibit the enzymatic activity of NA, thus slowing down the release of progeny virus from infected cells.

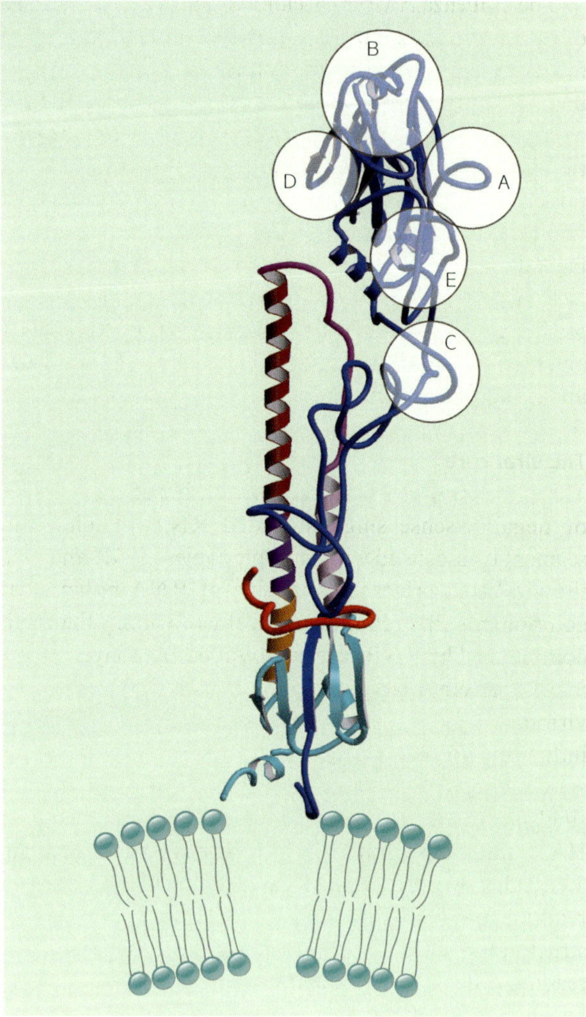

Figure 7. The location of the five major antigenic epitopes, A–E, on the HA1 subunit of the influenza virus haemagglutinin.[13] In the intact HA trimer, epitope D is not exposed and thus may not be involved in antibody induction. This figure was produced as explained in the caption to Figure 6.

The influenza A virus envelope contains a small number of copies of a third integral membrane protein, M2, which forms a tetramer with ion channel activity.[17–19] M2 is involved in the infection process by modulating the pH within virions, weakening the interaction between the viral ribonucleoproteins (RNPs) and the M1 protein. M2 is the target for the anti-influenza drugs amantadine and rimantadine.[20] Influenza B viruses also contain a similarly limited number of copies of the integral membrane protein NB.[17] This protein may well be a functional homologue of the M2 protein of the A viruses, but it is not inhibited by amantadine and rimantadine. Thus, these antiviral drugs are not effective against influenza B (see also pp. 152–165).

The viral core

The influenza A or B virus genome consists of eight strands of negative-sense single-stranded RNA.[1] Each RNA segment is associated with multiple copies of NP, and with the viral transcriptase consisting of RNA polymerase components PB1, PB2 and PA, thus forming the RNP complex.[21] The RNPs are surrounded by a layer of the matrix protein, M1. With approximately 3000 copies per virion, M1 is the most abundant structural protein of influenza virus.[1]

RNA segments 1–6 of influenza A viruses encode a single protein each.[1] For example, segment 4 encodes the HA, segment 5 NP and segment 6 the NA protein. Segment 7 encodes two proteins, M1 and M2, with overlapping reading frames. Likewise, segment 8 encodes the non-structural proteins NS1 and NS2, again with superimposed reading frames. Even though it was originally thought to be absent from virus particles (hence the name non-structural), NS2 has subsequently been identified in low copy numbers in virions. NS1 is not present in virions, but it is abundant in infected cells. Table 2 presents a survey of the RNA segments and the corresponding gene products of influenza A viruses.

Influenza A virus RNA segments and the proteins they encode

RNA segment (no. of nucleotides)	Gene product (no. of amino acids)	Molecules per virion
1 (2341)	Polymerase PB2 (759)	30–60
2 (2341)	Polymerase PB1 (757)	30–60
3 (2233)	Polymerase PA (716)	30–60
4 (1778)	Haemagglutinin (566)	500
5 (1565)	Nucleoprotein (498)	1000
6 (1413)	Neuraminidase (454)	100
7 (1027)	Matrix protein M1 (252) Matrix protein M2 (97)	3000 20–60
8 (890)	Non-structural protein NS1 (230) Non-structural protein NS2 (121)	– 130–200

Table 2. Influenza A virus RNA segments and the proteins they encode. Influenza A viruses have eight gene segments encoding 10 different proteins, segments 7 and 8 encoding two proteins each. Adapted from Lamb RA, Krug RM. *Orthomyxoviridae*: the viruses and their replication. In: Knipe DM, Howley PM, Griffin DE *et al*., editors. Fields *Virology*, 4th edn. Lippincott Williams & Wilkins, 2001; pp. 1487–1531[1] with permission from Lippincott Williams & Wilkins.

Virus replication

Receptor binding and cell entry

As indicated above, influenza viruses bind to sialic acid residues on glycoproteins or glycolipids on the host cell surface.[9] In humans, the primary targets for the virus are epithelial cells in the upper and lower respiratory tract. Cell binding of the virus occurs through the receptor-binding pocket at the distal tip of the HA molecule (Figure 6). The fine specificity of HA's receptor binding depends on the nature of the glycosidic linkage between the terminal sialic acid and the penultimate galactose residue on the receptor.[22] Human influenza viruses preferentially bind to sialic acids attached to galactose in an α2,6 configuration, whereas avian viruses have a preference for sialic acids attached to galactose in an α2,3 linkage.[23] This difference is thought to be the basis for the very inefficient transmission of avian influenza viruses to humans. Pigs, on the other hand, have receptors with either type of linkage between sialic acid and galactose, and thus are readily susceptible to infection with either human or avian viruses.[23] Co-infection of pigs with different influenza viruses is considered one mechanism by which new influenza viruses with pandemic potential may arise (see also pp. 45–67).

Receptor binding initiates uptake of the virus through so-called receptor-mediated endocytosis. In this process, virus particles are engulfed by the host cell plasma membrane (Figure 8). The vesicles thus formed subsequently fuse with intracellular compartments called endosomes, as a result of which the virus is delivered to the endosomal lumen.[24–26] Receptor-mediated endocytosis is not specific for uptake of viruses. In fact, it is a general mechanism by which cells internalize macromolecular complexes, including nutrients such as lipoproteins. Substances taken up by endocytosis, having traversed the endosomal cell compartment, generally end up in lysosomes, where they are degraded by hydrolytic enzymes. The influenza virus genome, however, escapes degradation; through fusion of the viral envelope with the endosomal membrane, it gains access to the cell cytosol.

Membrane fusion and uncoating of the viral core

It is the low pH inside the endosomes (pH 5–6), maintained by proton pumps within the endosomal membrane, that triggers the fusion reaction between the viral envelope and the endosomal membrane.[24,27] This is a key step in the viral

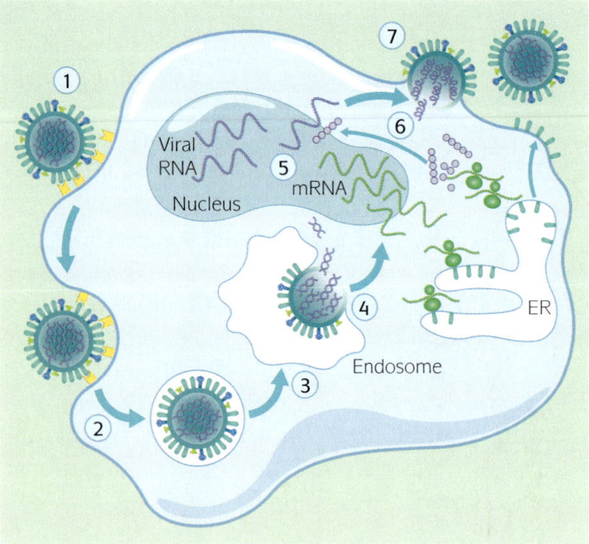

Figure 8. Life cycle of influenza virus. (1) Binding of the virus to a sialic acid-containing receptor. (2) Engulfment of the virus by the cell plasma membrane and formation of an endocytic vesicle. (3) Delivery of the virus to the endosomal cell compartment. (4) Fusion of the viral membrane with the membrane of the endosome, induced by the mildly acidic pH in the endosomal lumen. (5) Delivery of viral RNA to the nucleus, synthesis of messenger RNA (mRNA) and viral RNA replication. (6) Synthesis of viral protein components in the cell cytosol (internal proteins) and endoplasmic reticulum (ER) (membrane proteins). (7) Assembly and budding of progeny viruses. Adapted with kind permission of Linda Stannard.

infection mechanism. At low pH, a major conformational change in the HA spike is induced. This conformational change results in movement of the fusion peptide sequences of HA2, previously buried within the stem of the HA trimer, to the distal tip of the HA spike, allowing their insertion into the target membrane (Figure 9).[28,29] Subsequently, a complex process of bending of the trimer takes place promoted by the formation of a stable coiled

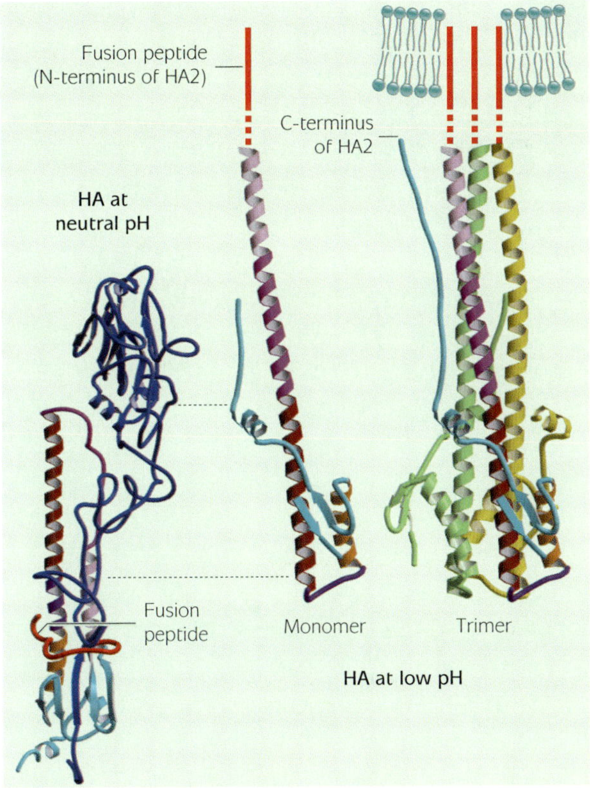

Figure 9. Conformational changes in the viral HA occuring at the pH of membrane fusion. The figure shows an HA monomer at neutral pH (left) and the low-pH form of HA2 both as a monomer and as a trimer (right). The long α-helices are represented in equivalent positions. As a result of the acid-induced conformational change in the molecule, the HA2 fusion peptides move upwards by about 10 nm to the tip of the trimer, such that they may insert into the endosomal membrane. Then the protein folds, while inducing membrane fusion, and the fusion peptide and the C-terminal membrane anchor, ultimately ending up in the same fused membrane. This figure was produced by André van Eerde (University of Groningen), using MOLSCRIPT, on the basis of co-ordinate files from the Protein Data Bank, codes 3HMG and 1HTM. Bullough PA *et al*. Structure of influenza haemagglutinin at the pH of membrane fusion. *Nature* 1994; **371**: 37–43.[29]

coil structure consisting of heptad repeat regions close to the fusion peptide and the transmembrane anchor of

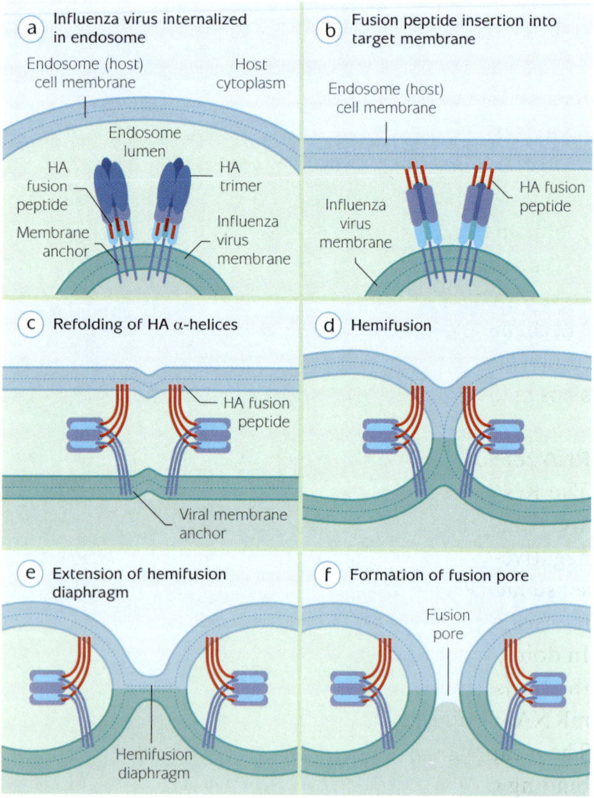

Figure 10. Hypothetical mechanism of HA-mediated fusion between the influenza virus membrane and the endosomal membrane, involving the formation of a hemifusion diaphragm. The key step in the fusion process is the relocation of the fusion peptides of HA2 to the tip of the HA trimer such that they can penetrate the endosomal membrane (step b); this step is triggered by the low pH in the endosomal lumen. Adapted from Cross KJ *et al*. Mechanisms of cell entry by influenza virus. *Exp Rev Molec Med*, 6 August 2001 (http://www-ermm.cbcu.cam.ac.uk/01003453h.htm) with permission from Cambridge University Press.

HA2.[30] Thus, the two ends of HA2 inserted into the apposed membranes are brought together. This then triggers merging of the two membranes, through which the viral core gains direct access to the cytosol of the cell (Figures 9 and 10).

The release of the viral RNPs from the endosome into the cytoplasm is facilitated by acidification of the viral interior prior to the fusion step. This acidification is mediated by the M2 proton channel in the viral envelope mentioned above.[17,20,31] After exposure of the virus to pH 5–6 within the lumen of the endosome, protons flow into the viral interior, weakening interaction of the M1 protein layer with the viral envelope and the RNPs. Blocking of the M2 channel with amantadine slows the dissociation of M1 from RNPs and the viral membrane, inhibiting subsequent steps in the viral life cycle (see pp. 152–165).[17,20,32]

RNA replication and translation

The RNP complexes released into the host cell cytosol are transported to the nucleus (Figure 8). Here, the negative-sense viral RNAs are transcribed to positive-sense messenger RNAs (mRNAs) by the transcriptase (consisting of PB1, PB2 and PA) carried with the RNPs.[1] In doing so, in a process referred to as "cap snatching", the transcriptase steals short cap regions from cellular mRNAs as primers for initiation of viral mRNA synthesis. These cap regions are subsequently required for efficient binding of ribosomes to the mRNA. Cap snatching by the viral transcriptase thus inhibits the synthesis of cellular proteins in favour of production of viral components. The mRNAs are transported back to the cell cytosol and translated into protein.

The negative-sense viral RNAs also serve as templates for production of exact positive-sense RNA copies (cRNA), which in turn direct the synthesis of multiple new copies of negative-sense viral RNAs. These genomic segments are transported back to the cell's cytosol for assembly into new virus particles.

Synthesis of the viral envelope proteins HA, NA and M2 starts in the cytosol, but already during synthesis, the growing polypeptide chains are transported into the endoplasmic reticulum (ER), where the proteins are folded and assembled into trimers and tetramers (Figure 8).[33,34] Also, in the ER, glycosylation of HA and NA is initiated. Subsequently, the proteins are transported through the Golgi apparatus and the trans-Golgi network (TGN) to the plasma membrane of the cell. Along this pathway, several modifications are introduced, including the formation of disulphide linkages and modification of the oligosaccharide side chains. Since the pH inside the TGN is mildly acidic, a premature fusion-activating conformational change in HA would likely be induced, had the virus not developed a protection mechanism against this. It so happens that M2, which is abundantly expressed in infected cells, through its proton channel activity transiently neutralizes the pH within the TGN, such that HA may transit safely to the cell surface.[17,20] This represents a second important function of the M2 protein, besides its role in viral entry and uncoating discussed above.

Synthesis and folding of viral core proteins occur entirely in the cytosol. NP and the RNA polymerase components interact with newly synthesized viral RNA to form RNPs. The M1 protein starts to interact with the C-terminal domains of HA and NA on the cell plasma membrane, forming patches with a high density of HA and NA, excluding cellular plasma membrane proteins. Subsequently, newly formed RNPs interact actively with the M1 lining at these patches (Figure 8). This interaction efficiently prevents re-entry of RNPs into the nucleus.

Assembly and release of new viral particles

After attachment of RNPs to M1 on the inner half of the cell plasma membranes, in an intriguing process of budding, new virus particles are assembled (Figure 8). In polarized epithelial cells, this process occurs exclusively on the apical side of the cells, HA and NA being sorted to this "exterior" surface of the cells' plasma membrane.[35] As a result, progeny virus is released back to the airways and not to the systemic circulation.

It has long been thought that the packaging of RNPs into new virions occurs in an entirely random fashion. Thus, many non-infectious virus particles would be formed with an incomplete set of RNA segments, whereas just a minority of particles would contain the full complement of the proper eight RNA segments. More recent observations indicate, however, that packaging of RNPs is not a random process, but rather favours the formation of infectious virus particles with all eight RNA segments required for infection.[36] However, also with packaging of RNPs occurring in a directed fashion, upon co-infection of a cell with two influenza viruses from different origins (e.g. avian and human), this assembly process may result in mixing of RNA segments of the two different viruses into a new virus with an altered genetic make-up. This mixing of gene segments, referred to as genetic reassortment, is one mechanism by which new influenza viruses with pandemic potential may arise (see also pp. 45–67).

After budding, the new virions are still attached to the cell surface through interaction of the HA with sialic acid residues on cellular glycoproteins or glycolipids. It is now that the viral NA cleaves the sialic acid, thus releasing the virions from the host cell's surface,[15] allowing them to spread further throughout the respiratory tract. Antibodies directed against the NA or neuraminidase inhibitors can block neuraminidase activity, thus preventing release and spreading of the new viruses (see also pp. 152–165). This also explains why antibodies against NA, like the neuraminidase inhibitors, do not neutralize virus infection, but rather aid in ameliorating the infection process.

The entire process of viral infection seriously disrupts the normal physiology of the cell. This, in the case of influenza, as with many other acute lytic viral infections, eventually leads to cell death. Cell death results in desquamation of the respiratory epithelium as one aspect of influenza pathogenesis (see also pp. 86–106). However, cell lysis does not occur until the cell has produced many thousands of new virus particles.

Cleavage activation of HA and viral pathogenicity

As mentioned above, in the infected cell, HA is synthesized as a single polypeptide chain (HA0). Cleavage of HA0 into HA1 and HA2 is a prerequisite for the expression of HA's membrane fusion activity, later on when newly formed virus particles enter new target cells. Thus, cleavage of HA0 is essential for viral infectivity.[1,11,12,28,29] In human influenza viruses, cleavage is thought to occur extracellularly, after HA has been incorporated in virus particles.[37] Cleavage occurs at a single arginine residue at the clip site. The enzyme responsible for cleavage, a trypsin-like protease, is probably released from Clara cells in the respiratory epithelium. Since the tissue distribution of this enzyme is limited, human influenza viruses do not normally spread beyond the respiratory tract.

For avian influenza viruses, the situation is somewhat different and appears to be closely related to the pathogenicity of these viruses in birds.[37,38] HAs of non-virulent, or low-pathogenicity, avian influenza viruses have a single basic cleavage site similar to that in HAs of human viruses, restricting the spread of these viruses. On the other hand, HAs of highly pathogenic avian influenza viruses ("fowl plague" viruses) appear to have a multibasic cleavage site, as a result of which these HAs can be cleaved by intracellular furin-like proteases, in a process that occurs just before the HA molecules reach the surface of the infected cell. Since furin-like proteases are present in virtually every cell type, avian viruses with HAs containing a multibasic cleavage site can easily spread throughout the body, often causing a fatal systemic infection.

It is not clear whether the presence of a multibasic cleavage site in HA0 also represents an important determinant of viral pathogenicity in humans.[37] The HA of the extrememely pathogenic Spanish flu virus, which caused one of the most devastating pandemics in the history of mankind, does not have the multibasic cleavage site.[39] On the other hand, human infections with the highly pathogenic H5N1 avian influenza virus, which does have the multibasic cleavage site in its HA, exhibited very high case-fatality rates, with six deaths from 18 confirmed cases in Hong Kong in 1997 and 23 deaths from 34 infections in Vietnam and Thailand in 2004. This suggests that the presence of a multibasic cleavage site in HA may be a determinant of systemic spread and viral pathogenicity in humans, although other factors are probably involved as well.

References

1. Lamb RA, Krug RM. Orthomyxoviridae: the viruses and their replication. In: Knipe DM, Howley PM, Griffin DE *et al.*, editors. Fields *Virology*, 4th edn. Lippincott Williams & Wilkins, 2001; pp. 1487–1531.

2. Wright PF, Webster RG. Orthomyxoviruses. In: Knipe DM, Howley PM, Griffin DE *et al.*, editors. Fields *Virology*, 4th edn. Lippincott Williams & Wilkins, 2001; pp. 1533–1579.

3. Moser MR, Bender TR, Margolis HS *et al.* An outbreak of influenza aboard a commercial airliner. *Am J Epidemiol* 1979; **110**: 1–6.

4. Hinshaw VS, Webster RG, Bean WJ, Sriram G. The ecology of influenza viruses in ducks and analysis of influenza viruses with monoclonal antibodies. *Comp Immunol Microbiol Infect Dis* 1980; **3**: 155–164.

5. Osterhaus ADME, Rimmelzwaan GF, Martina BE, Bestebroer TM, Fouchier RAM. Influenza B virus in seals. *Science* 2000; **288**: 1051–1053.

6. WHO Memorandum. A revised system for nomenclature of influenza viruses. *Bull World Health Org* 1980; **58**: 585–591.

7. Ruigrok RWH. Structure of influenza A, B and C viruses. In: Nicholson KG, Webster RG, Hay AJ, editors. *Textbook of Influenza*. Blackwell Science, 1998; pp. 29–42.

8. Steinhauer DA, Wharton SA. Structure and function of the haemagglutinin. In: Nicholson KG, Webster RG, Hay AJ,

editors. *Textbook of Influenza*. Blackwell Science, 1998; pp. 54–64.

9. Colman PM. Structure and function of the neuraminidase. In: Nicholson KG, Webster RG, Hay AJ, editors. *Textbook of Influenza*. Blackwell Science, 1998; pp. 65–73.

10. Varghese JN, Laver WG, Colman PM. Structure of the influenza virus glycoprotein antigen neuraminidase at 2.9 Å resolution. *Nature* 1983; **303**: 35–40.

11. Wilson IA, Skehel JJ, Wiley DC. Structure of the haemagglutinin membrane glycoprotein of influenza virus at 3 Å resolution. *Nature* 1981; **289**: 366–373.

12. Skehel JJ, Wiley DC. Receptor binding and membrane fusion in virus entry: the influenza hemagglutinin. *Annu Rev Biochem* 2000; **69**: 531–569.

13. Wiley DC, Wilson IA, Skehel JJ. Structural identification of the antibody-binding sites of Hong Kong influenza haemagglutinin and their involvement in antigenic variation. *Nature* 1981; **289**: 373–378.

14. Hirst GK. Adsorption of influenza haemagglutinins and virus by red blood cells. *J Exp Med* 1942; **76**: 195–209.

15. Palese P, Compans RW. Inhibition of influenza virus replication in tissue culture by 2-deoxy-2,3-dehydro-N-trifluoroacetylneuraminic acid (FANA): mechanism of action. *J Gen Virol* 1976; **33**: 159–163.

16. Von Itzstein M, Wu WY, Kok GB *et al*. Rational design of potent sialidase-based inhibitors of influenza virus replication. *Nature* 1993; **363**: 418–423.

17. Hay AJ. Functional properties of the virus ion channels. In: Nicholson KG, Webster RG, Hay AJ, editors. *Textbook of Influenza*. Blackwell Science, 1998; pp. 74–81.

18. Lamb RA, Zebedee SL, Richardson CD. Influenza virus M2 protein is an integral membrane protein expressed on the infected-cell surface. *Cell* 1985; **40**: 627–633.

19. Zebedee SL, Lamb RA. Influenza A virus M2 protein: monoclonal antibody restriction of virus growth and detection of M2 in virions. *J Virol* 1988; **62**: 2762–2772.

20. Hay AJ. The action of adamantanamines against influenza A viruses: inhibition of the M2 channel protein. *Semin Virol* 1992; **3**: 21–30.

21. Duesberg PH. Distinct subunits of the ribonucleoprotein of influenza virus. *J Molec Biol* 1969; **42**: 485–499.

22. Weis W, Brown JH, Cusack S *et al*. Structure of the influenza virus haemagglutinin complexed with its receptor, sialic acid. *Nature* 1988; **333**: 426–431.

23. Ito T, Couceiro JN, Kelm S *et al*. Molecular basis for the generation in pigs of influenza A viruses with pandemic potential. *J Virol* 1998; **72**: 7367–7373.

24. Matlin KS, Reggio H, Helenius A, Simons K. Infectious entry pathway of influenza virus in a canine kidney cell line. *J Cell Biol* 1981; **91**: 601–613.

25. Marsh M, Helenius A. Virus entry into animal cells. *Adv Virus Res* 1989; **36**: 107–151.

26. Smith AE, Helenius A. How viruses enter animal cells. *Science* 2004; **304**: 237–242.

27. Stegmann T, Morselt HW, Scholma J, Wilschut J. Fusion of influenza virus in an intracellular acidic compartment measured by fluorescence dequenching. *Biochim Biophys Acta* 1987; **904**: 165–170.

28. Kim Carr CM, Kim PS. A spring-loaded mechanism for the conformational change of influenza hemagglutinin. *Cell* 1993; **73**: 823–832.

29. Bullough PA, Hughson FM, Skehel JJ, Wiley DC. Structure of influenza haemagglutinin at the pH of membrane fusion. *Nature* 1994; **371**: 37–43.

30. Chen J, Skehel JJ, Wiley DC. N- and C-terminal residues combine in the fusion–pH influenza hemagglutinin HA(2) subunit to form an N cap that terminates the triple-stranded coiled coil. *Proc Natl Acad Sci USA* 1999; **96**: 8967–8972.

31. Helenius A. Unpacking the incoming influenza virus. *Cell* 1992; **69**: 577–578.

32. Bron R, Kendal AP, Klenk HD, Wilschut J. Role of the M2 protein in influenza virus membrane fusion: effects of amantadine and monensin on fusion kinetics. *Virology* 1993; **195**: 808–811.

33. Braakman I, Hoover-Litty H, Wagner KR, Helenius A. Folding of influenza hemagglutinin in the endoplasmic reticulum. *J Cell Biol* 1991; **114**: 401–411.

34. Doms RW, Lamb RA, Rose JK, Helenius A. Folding and assembly of viral membrane proteins. *Virology* 1993; **193**: 545–562.

35. Rodriguez-Boulan E, Sabatini DD. Asymmetric budding of viruses in epithelial monlayers: a model system for study of epithelial polarity. *Proc Natl Acad Sci USA* 1978; **75**: 5071–5075.

36. Fujii Y, Goto H, Watanabe T, Yoshida T, Kawaoka Y. Selective incorporation of influenza virus RNA segments into virions. *Proc Natl Acad Sci USA* 2003; **100**: 2002–2007.

37. Steinhauer DA. Role of hemagglutinin cleavage for the pathogenicity of influenza virus. *Virology* 1999; **258**: 1–20.

38. Klenk H-D, Garten W. Host cell proteases controlling virus pathogenicity. *Trends Microbiol* 1994; **2**: 39–43.

39. Reid AH, Fanning TG, Hultin JV, Taubenberger JK. Origin and evolution of the 1918 "Spanish" influenza virus hemagglutinin gene. *Proc Natl Acad Sci USA* 1999; **96**: 1651–1656.

Antigenic Drift and Shift: Epidemic and Pandemic Influenza

The influenza viruses continuously undergo antigenic variation.[1] It is this quality that allows them to evade the immune system of the host – immune responses mounted against earlier forms of the virus are less effective or completely ineffective against newer variants. Since the viral surface glycoprotein HA is the antigen against which virus-neutralizing antibodies are directed (pp. 68–85), it is primarily the antigenic variation of HA that is responsible for the immune escape of the influenza virus. However, other viral antigens also undergo significant variation, and thus contribute to the evasion of the immune defence of the host as well.[2] The antigenic variation of influenza viruses forms the primary basis for the occurrence of annual influenza epidemics and occasional pandemics. Also, it necessitates regular updates of the composition of the influenza vaccines (see pp. 124–151).

There are two main mechanisms by which influenza A viruses change their antigenic properties. These are commonly referred to as "antigenic drift" and "antigenic shift".[1] Antigenic drift occurs as a result of continuous mutation of the RNA genome of the virus due to errors that are made during the RNA replication process. As a result, amino acid changes in the viral proteins arise, including substitutions in the antigenic epitopes of HA. Virus variants with such substitutions have a selective advantage over the original virus, if they are no longer or less efficiently countered by the pre-existing immunity of the host.

Occasionally, an entirely new influenza A virus subtype of avian origin emerges in the human population. This is referred to as antigenic shift. Since there is no immunity whatsoever to the new subtype in the population, this forms the scenario for a pandemic outbreak of influenza. Antigenic shift may be the result of direct transmission of an avian virus to humans. There are reasons to believe that such a direct introduction of an avian influenza virus into the human population caused the pandemic of Spanish flu in 1918.[3–5] A human influenza virus may also acquire just a number of genes from an avian virus, pigs or humans serving as a "mixing vessel". Such a process of scrambling of genes might result in the formation of a new virus with most of the properties of a normal human influenza virus, yet having a new HA subtype on its surface to which the population is immunologically naive.[1] For example, the 1957 Asian flu and 1968 Hong Kong flu viruses arose as a result of an exchange of genes between avian and human influenza viruses.

Three major influenza pandemics struck the world in the 20th century. By far the most devastating pandemic was that of the Spanish flu, which hit at the end of the First World War. It spread across the globe in three consecutive waves in 1918–19, killing at least 40 million people, thus causing more victims than the 1914–18 war itself. There is no doubt that there will be other pandemics in the future.[6,7] Having its reservoir among migratory waterfowl, influenza is a non-eradicable zoonosis that will continue to affect humans. The recent outbreaks of highly pathogenic avian influenza with occasional transmissions to humans, causing infections with very high case-fatality rates, should serve as a warning that a new pandemic is just a matter of time. Accordingly, the WHO is urging individual countries to be aware of the need to start formal influenza pandemic preparedness planning as soon as possible.

Key Messages

- Influenza viruses continuously change their antigenic properties through "antigenic drift" and "antigenic shift".
- Antigenic drift is due to accumulation of mutations in antigenic epitopes of viral antigens. As a result, pre-existing antibodies against the viral HA no longer neutralize newer drift variants of the virus.
- Antigenic drift of HA is the cause of recurrent annual influenza epidemics. It necessitates repeated vaccination of target groups and regular updates of the vaccine composition.
- The natural reservoir of influenza A viruses is among wild aquatic birds. All 15 subtypes of HA and all nine subtypes of NA have been identified in waterfowl.
- Antigenic shift implies that an influenza A virus with a new HA subtype is introduced into the human population. This may occur by (i) genetic reassortment between an avian and a human virus, (ii) direct transmission of an avian virus from birds to humans, or (iii) reintroduction of an "old" strain into the population.
- Antigenic shift is the cause of occasional global outbreaks of influenza (pandemics). These arise primarily because of a total lack of immunity against the new virus subtype in the population.
- Since the reservoir of influenza A viruses is among wild birds and avian viruses do occasionally cross the species barrier to humans, influenza is a non-eradicable disease and pandemics will continue to occur.
- Intensive surveillance of influenza activity among birds (and other species, including humans) is required for optimal pandemic preparedness.

Antigenic drift

Nature of antigenic drift

The replication of viral RNA in an infected host cell is an error-prone process, much more so than the replication of DNA. One reason for this is the lack of so-called proofreading mechanisms in the replication of RNA. As a result, the error rate of influenza virus RNA replication is approximately one in 100,000 nucleotides.[8] Considering that the size of the entire influenza virus genome is about 14,000 nucleotides, this implies that many new viral RNA genome copies will contain one or more mutations. While many of these mutations will be silent or generate stop codons, others will result in amino acid substitutions in the translated proteins, which may give the new variant an advantage over the parent virus. Antigenic drift of HA occurs as a result of accumulation of point mutations in the antigenic domains (epitopes) of HA1 (see Figure 7). Selective advantage for the new variants in this case arises because these variants are no longer inhibited by the immunity of the host.

Antigenic drift is a gradual process. Mutations may arise in one epitope of HA while other epitopes remain unchanged. Thus, depending on the nature of the mutation, the new strain may still be partially recognized by the immune defence of the host. This gradual change is illustrated in Table 3, which shows that drift variants of the 1968 Hong Kong pandemic virus gradually lose the ability to cross-react with an antiserum against the original virus, while antisera against increasingly distant drift viruses no longer cross-react with the 1968 strain.[1] Antigenic drift may be so pronounced that the new variant virus is not even partially recognized by the antibodies of the host. In that case, the drift virus may behave like a "shift" virus with pandemic potential.[9]

Table 3. Antigenic drift of influenza H3N2 virus from 1968 to 1997. The table provides haemagglutination–inhibition titres (see pp.124–151) of ferret antisera against drift variants of the H3N2 virus. Reproduced from Wright PF, Webster RG. Orthomyxoviruses. In: Knipe DM, Howley PM, Griffin DE *et al.*, editors. Fields *Virology*, 4th edn. Lippincott Williams & Wilkins, 2001; pp. 1533–1579[1] with permission from Lippincott Williams & Wilkins.

Antigenic drift of influenza H3N2 virus from 1968 to 1997

	Reference ferret antisera									
Strain designation	HK/68 1.	ENG/72 2.	VIC/75 3.	TEX/77 4.	BANG/79 5.	PHIL/82 6.	MISS/85 7.	SHN/87 8.	BEI/89 9.	BEI/92 10.
1. A/Hong Kong/01/68	*2560*	1280	40	5	5	5	10	10	5	5
2. A/England/42/72	320	*1280*	80	20	5	5	5	5	5	5
3. A/Victoria/03/75	5	80	*320*	40	10	20	10	5	5	5
4. A/Texas/01/77	5	80	160	*1280*	160	320	320	10	10	5
5. A/Bangkok/01/79	5	5	80	640	*640*	640	640	20	10	5
6. A/Philippines/02/82	5	5	10	40	40	*320*	160	10	10	5
7. A/Mississippi/01/85	5	5	40	160	80	640	*640*	40	20	20
8. A/Shanghai/11/87	5	5	5	5	5	5	80	*320*	160	20
9. A/Beijing/353/89	5	5	5	5	5	5	5	160	*320*	40
10. A/Beijing/32/92	5	5	5	5	5	5	10	20	80	*640*
11. A/Johannesburg/33/94	5	5	5	5	5	5	5	10	20	160
12. A/Nanchang/933/95	5	5	5	5	5	5	5	5	10	20
13. A/Sydney05/97	5	5	5	5	5	5	5	5	5	5

Influenza epidemics

Despite their annual seasonal character, influenza epidemics are unpredictable.[7] When precisely they will start, how long they will last and how virulent they will be are questions that are difficult to answer in advance. The severity of an epidemic in any given year is a subtle interplay between the waning immunity in the population, the extent of antigenic drift of the virus and the intrinsic virulence of the new virus variant.

While in tropical countries influenza may be present all year round, epidemics in temperate regions occur almost exclusively in the winter months, from November to April in the northern hemisphere and from May to October in the southern hemisphere. However, there is considerable variation in the onset and duration of epidemics, as illustrated in Figure 11. It is not clear why there is this seasonal regularity in the occurrence of annual influenza outbreaks. One reason is thought to be crowding of people in closed spaces with poor ventilation. For example, spreading of the virus may be facilitated in schools – there is evidence that schoolchildren in particular play a prominent role in the transmission of influenza.[10]

Regular update of vaccine composition

The antigenic drift of influenza virus necessitates regular updates of the composition of the influenza vaccine. Obviously, a close match of the virus strains in the vaccine and the strains subsequently circulating in the winter season is of key importance for the protective efficacy of the vaccine. As discussed in more detail on pages 124–151, current inactivated influenza vaccines contain three virus strains (two A strains and one B strain), included in the vaccine on annual recommendation by the WHO. This recommendation is based on intensive surveillance of new viruses (see below), such that an optimally informed selection of vaccine strains can be made. In general, the system of selection of vaccine virus strains works quite well. However, the prediction of which viruses will be circulating in the next winter season has an inherent degree

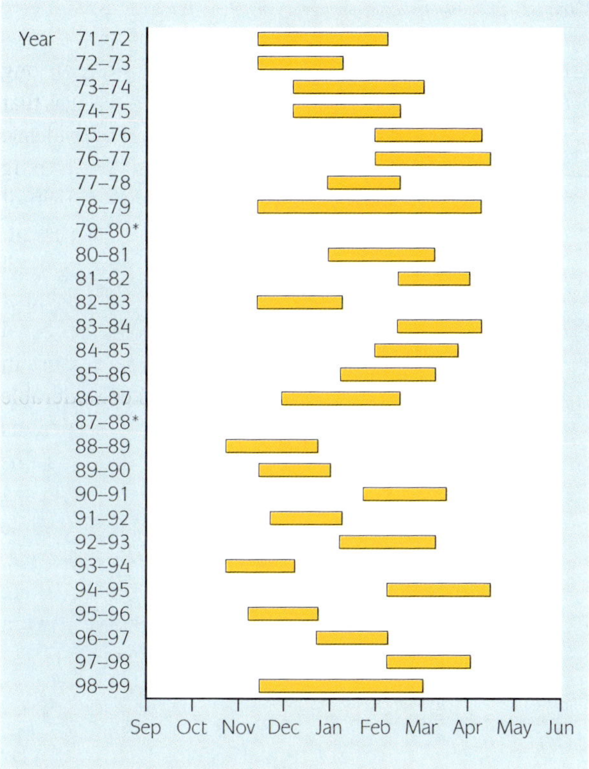

Figure 11. Onset and duration of influenza epidemics in the Netherlands, 1971–1999. Courtesy of Solvay Pharmaceuticals, Weesp, The Netherlands.

of uncertainty. This implies that occasional mismatches do occur. In these cases, the influenza vaccination may have limited efficacy, but this should not discourage people in target groups to take the vaccination in the next season.

Antigenic shift

Currently available information suggests that the natural reservoirs for influenza A viruses are aquatic birds.[3,11–15] All 15 HA and nine NA subtypes have been identified in birds (see pp. 23–44). Occasionally, a new influenza virus subtype is introduced into the human population, in a process referred to as antigenic shift.[16] There are multiple ways by which such new human virus subtypes may arise (Figure 12),

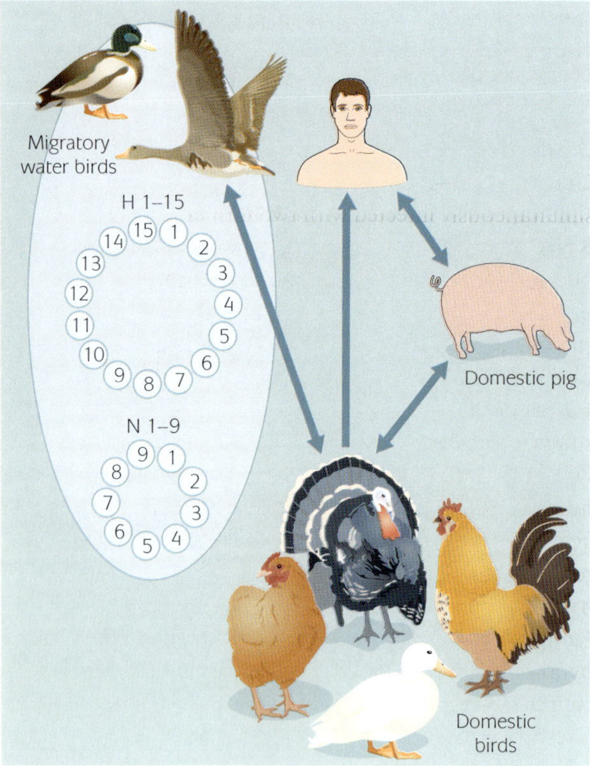

Figure 12. Origin of antigenic shift and pandemic influenza. The natural reservoir of influenza A viruses is among migratory aquatic birds. A virus with a new HA subtype may be introduced into the human population by direct transmission of an avian virus to humans or by genetic reassortment between an avian and a human virus. Adapted from Nicholson KG *et al*. Influenza. *Lancet* 2003; **362**: 1733–1745[7] with permission from Elsevier.

and it is likely that each has played a role in the influenza pandemics of the 20th century. First, a circulating human influenza virus may exchange a number of gene segments with an avian virus in a process of so-called genetic reassortment.[17] Second, an avian virus may be transmitted directly to humans without an intermediate reassortment step.[3,18–20] Third, it is also possible that an "old" human virus, which has circulated before, is reintroduced into the human population.[21]

Genetic reassortment

Genetic reassortment occurs when a host cell is simultaneously infected with two influenza A viruses. The RNA segments from both viruses are replicated in the nucleus of the cell. During the reassembly of new virus particles (see pp. 23–44), the RNA segments from the two strains can get mixed together and a third "new" viral strain can be produced with a unique genetic make-up.

As illustrated in Figure 13, the 1957 Asian H2N2 virus subtype obtained its HA, NA, and PB1 genes from an avian virus and the other fives genes from the circulating H1N1 human strain.[11,12,22] Likewise, the Hong Kong H3N2 virus acquired its HA and PB1 genes from an avian virus, but retained the NA plus five other genes from the circulating human virus. It is remarkable that the H3 of the Hong Kong virus differed in only seven amino acids from its hypothetical avian ancestor virus, providing very strong support for the concept that the Hong Kong virus arose as a result of genetic reassortment.[23]

It has long been thought that genetic reassortment would occur exclusively in pigs.[7,11,12,22] The pig provides an ideal "mixing vessel", since pigs are readily infectable by both human and avian influenza viruses due to the molecular nature of their sialic acid-containing receptors (see pp. 23–44). However, there is increasing evidence now that other species, including man (see below), might also serve as mixing vessels.

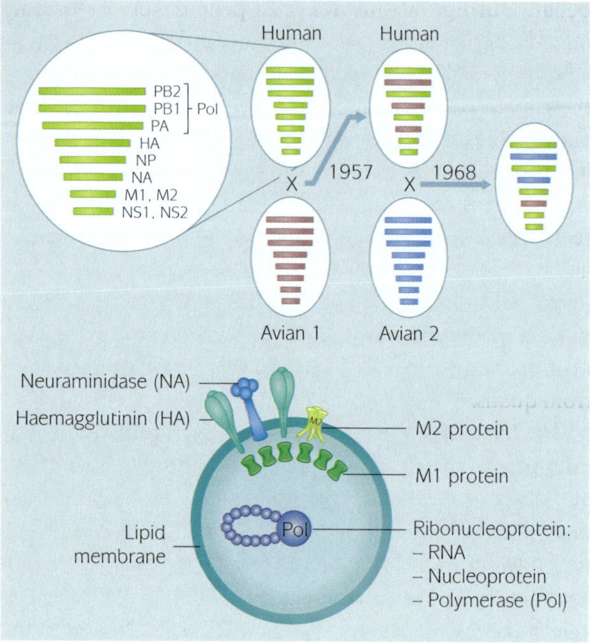

Figure 13. Genetic reassortment between human and avian influenza A viruses as the origin of the pandemic 1957 Asian flu and 1968 Hong Kong flu viruses. The segmented nature of the influenza virus genome facilitates reassortment. Pigs – which support the replication of both avian and human influenza A viruses – possibly serve as a "mixing vessel". The Asian H2N2 virus subtype obtained its HA, NA and PB1 genes from an avian virus. Likewise, the HA and PB1 genes of the Hong Kong H3N2 virus are of avian origin – the Hong Kong virus retained the NA gene plus five other genes from the circulating human virus. Adapted from Potter CW, editor. *Influenza (Perspectives in Medical Virology)*, 2003 with permission from Elsevier.

Direct transmission of avian viruses to humans

Rarely, an avian influenza virus is transmitted directly to humans without pigs serving as an intermediate host. It was not until the 1997 "bird flu" outbreak in Hong Kong that it was appreciated that such direct transmission could occur. During this outbreak, 18 people were reportedly infected with a highly pathogenic avian H5N1 virus, six of whom died.[3,18–20] The virus isolated from the victims had the same genetic make-up as the virus causing the epidemic among chickens in Hong Kong at the time, indicating that it was transmitted directly from chickens to humans.

The H5N1 bird flu virus was in fact a "multiple avian reassortant", which originated from an H5N1 reservoir in geese, reassorted before crossing to terrestrial poultry (especially chickens), and then probably acquired the internal protein genes and the NA gene through further reassortment with H9N2 and H6N1 viruses originating from quails.[24]

The bird flu outbreak in 1997 was the first documented example of a purely avian virus causing respiratory disease and deaths among humans.[3,18–20] Clearly, the H5N1 virus, once having crossed the species barrier to humans, replicated efficiently, killing one-third of the people with a confirmed H5N1 infection. Fortunately, there was no evidence for human-to-human transmission of the virus. Additional mutations or reassortment events are probably required to permit efficient human-to-human spread. Indeed, in 1997 it was feared that the avian H5N1 virus might reassort with a human influenza virus, with humans now serving as the mixing vessel. Such a reassortment might have created a new virulent virus capable of airborne human-to-human transmission.

Even without reassortment in humans, adaptation of an avian virus in the human host might give rise to a virus capable of human-to-human transmission, through mutation of the viral HA. There is evidence that the 1918 Spanish influenza virus had arisen in this manner.[3] Analysis of viral genes recovered from post-mortem lung tissue of victims of the pandemic has indicated that the HA was of avian origin.[4] Recent determination of the structure and receptor-binding properties of the 1918 HA confirms this and suggests that, by mutation of the receptor-binding site, the HA acquired the ability to interact with human α2,6-linked sialic acid receptors (see pp. 23–44), thus explaining the ability of the virus to spread efficiently from human to human.[5] Therefore, it is possible that an H1N1 avian virus entered the human population by direct transmission, similar to the recent transmissions seen with H5N1, and subsequently adapted to the human host through mutation of HA's receptor-binding properties.[3] Indeed, there is some evidence that the virus entered the human population several years before the pandemic.[3,4] While there is a close genetic relationship between the 1918 virus and the porcine A/Swine/Iowa/30 (H1N1) virus, this does not necessarily imply that the human virus originated in pigs. Rather, a precursor of the 1918 virus may have been transmitted from humans to pigs.[3]

Reintroduction of an old strain

A third way by which an antigenic shift may occur and a pandemic arise is reintroduction of an "old" strain into the human population. A virus could remain hidden – for example, in a frozen state such that little change would occur – and re-emerge as a pandemic virus when the immunity in the population to that virus has decreased. The appearance of the Russian flu (H1N1) in 1977 supports the idea of reintroduction of a previous strain. The virus turned out to be identical in all of its genes to the H1N1 virus that circulated before 1957 and caused a major epidemic in 1950.[21]

Influenza pandemics

Historic records indicate that influenza epidemics and pandemics have been among us for many centuries.[9,25] A report by Hippocrates describes an outbreak as early as 412 BC that could have been due to influenza. Several further accounts are suggestive of influenza outbreaks, but lack sufficient scientific substance to provide certainty. The first convincing report of an influenza pandemic describes an outbreak in 1580, which started in Asia in the summer, and then spread via Africa to Europe and finally to America.[26] In Britain it came in two waves, a pattern that

Definition of pandemic influenza
• A new influenza A virus emerges in the human population, with an HA subtype unrelated to the influenza viruses circulating immediately before the outbreak, such that it could not have arisen by mutation.
• Immunity to the new virus subtype is absent in a large proportion of the population.
• The virus is capable of spreading by person-to-person transmission; a high percentage of individuals is infected, causing increased morbidity and mortality.
• The infection spreads rapidly beyond its site of origin throughout the world.

Table 4. Definition of pandemic influenza. Adapted from Webster RG, Laver WG. Pandemic variation of influenza viruses. In: Kilbourne ED, editor. *The Influenza Viruses and Influenza*. Academic Press, 1975; pp. 269–314[16] with permission from Academic Press.

was also seen in many subsequent influenza pandemics. Other convincing accounts of influenza pandemics followed in the 18th and 19th centuries.[25]

A number of conditions must be satisfied in order for an outbreak of influenza to be classified as a "pandemic".[16] These are indicated in Table 4. Before the first isolation of the influenza virus from humans in 1933, the identification of influenza pandemics was based solely on epidemiological records and morbidity and mortality rates. However, both epidemiological data and molecular analysis of the new virus are required to identify a pandemic virus with certainty. The pandemics that occurred in the 20th century will be described in some detail below.

Pandemics of the past century

Figure 14 gives an overview of the influenza pandemics that occurred in the past century.[9,25,26] The most terrible outbreak was the Spanish flu in 1918, with an estimated

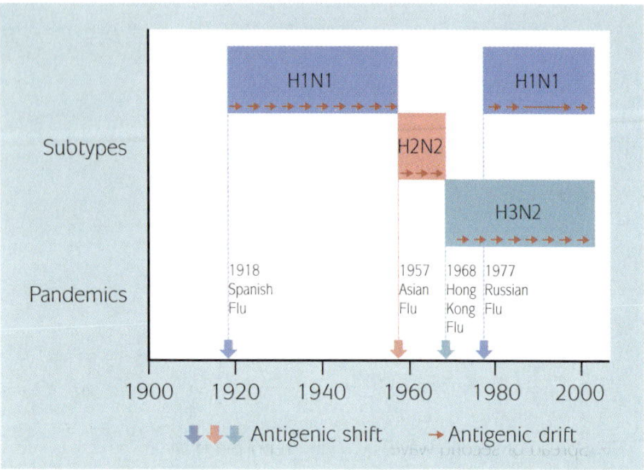

Figure 14. Influenza A viruses of the 20th century pandemics. The 1918 Spanish flu virus (H1N1) probably originated through direct transmission of an avian virus to man and further adaptation of this virus to the human host. The 1957 Asian (H2N2) and 1968 Hong Kong (H3N2) viruses were reassortants of avian and circulating human viruses (see Figure 13). The 1977 Russian flu virus was an old strain, reintroduced into the human population. Courtesy of Solvay Pharmaceuticals, Weesp, the Netherlands.

40 million deaths, justifying its description as "the last great plague of mankind".

1918 – Spanish flu (H1N1)

The Spanish flu first struck in March 1918 in the USA, with reports from Detroit, South Carolina and San Quentin Prison of outbreaks of an unusual respiratory disease that was associated with a disproportionate increase in deaths among young adults. The infection spread rapidly, crossing both the Atlantic and Pacific Oceans in a matter of months, killing many American soldiers during their voyage to Europe in the spring of 1918 (Figure 15). In Europe, initial infections were reported in Madrid in May 1918, hence the name "Spanish" flu. This first wave infected all the armies in Europe during May and June. After the initial wave there

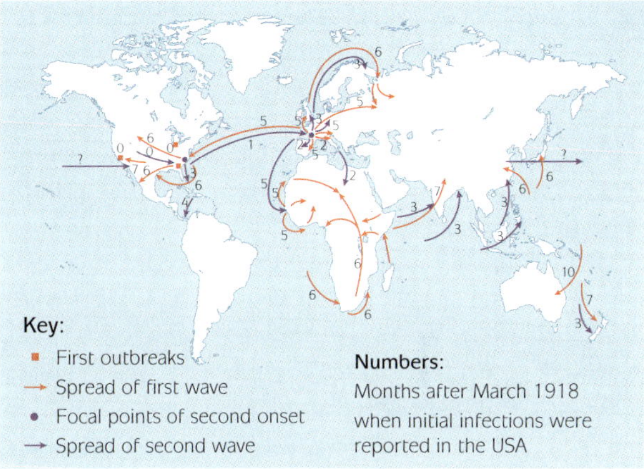

Figure 15. The 1918 Spanish flu pandemic. The origin of the Spanish influenza virus (H1N1) is unclear. First outbreaks were reported in the USA in March 1918. The infection rapidly spread to Europe, where its impact was particularly terrible, and further throughout the world. After the first wave in the spring of 1918, a second, more devastating wave followed in the fall of 1918 and a third wave in the spring of 1919. The pandemic killed over 40 million people. Adapted from Potter CW. Chronicle of influenza pandemics. In: Nicholson KG, Webster RG, Hay AJ, editors. *Textbook of Influenza*. Oxford: Blackwell Science, 1998; pp. 3–18[25] with permission from Blackwell Publishing.

was a sharp decline of infections in the summer of 1918, to be followed by a second, more severe, wave that peaked in the autumn of 1918, and a third wave in the spring of 1919, both associated with global spread of the infection. In just 10 months, 40 million people worldwide died, more than the total number of victims of the 1914–18 war.

The origin of the Spanish influenza is not clear. It may have been imported into the USA by migrant workers from China. It is equally possible that the pandemic originated in the USA. Indeed, the fact that the pandemic started with simultaneous outbreaks at three different locations in the USA supports this hypothesis.

1957 – Asian flu (H2N2)

The "Asian flu" originated in the Yunan Province of China in March 1957, spreading rapidly to South-East Asia and Japan, and subsequently in May to Australia, Indonesia and India, and during the summer to Europe, Africa, North and South America, and the Caribbean. In just 6 months, the pandemic had spanned the globe. A second wave occurred during the autumn of 1957. Altogether it affected some 40–50% of the population, with 25–30% experiencing clinical disease. Mortality was approximately 1/4000, occurring predominantly among the very young and the very old. The total death rate probably exceeded 1 million.

1968 – Hong Kong flu (H3N2)

This pandemic also originated in China, in July 1968, spreading to Hong Kong, where it peaked after only 2 weeks, causing a major outbreak of 500,000 cases, and receded completely after 6 weeks. By August, the infection had spread to Taiwan, the Philippines, Singapore and Vietnam, and by September to India, Iran and Australia. In that month the infection also entered North America via California, carried by troops returning from Vietnam. In the USA, the epidemic peaked in December. Altogether, 30–40% of the population were infected, causing 56,000 excess deaths. School absenteeism reached 50%. Compared to the earlier pandemics of the century, the Hong Kong flu was relatively mild; worldwide, the total death toll was approximately 500,000.

1977 – Russian flu (H1N1)

The outbreak of Russian flu first appeared in northen China in May 1977 and spread throughout Russia by December, and the rest of the world in 1978. As mentioned above, the virus was subsequently found to be virtually identical to one that had caused a human epidemic in 1950.[21] Consequently, most people over 23 years old possessed antibody to it. Thus, the pandemic was confined almost entirely to children and teenagers. Thankfully, the illness was quite mild and weekly attack rates at peak were about 13% in children 7–14 years old. Unlike the previous two pandemic viruses, this virus failed to replace the previously circulating influenza A virus and currently both H1N1 and H3N2 viruses circulate in humans.

Will there be a new pandemic?

There is no doubt that there will be influenza pandemics in the future.[3,7,13,14] It is not so much a matter of *whether* they will occur but rather *when* they will occur. All the ingredients for the formation of new influenza viruses with pandemic potential are there, particularly in China. As indicated above, the 1957 H2N2 and 1968 H3N2 viruses originated in China. It is thought that the ecological conditions in China are such that new viruses with pandemic potential may arise comparatively easily. These include the year-round circulation of influenza viruses, along with the dense populations of people, pigs and domestic poultry, often living in close proximity – conditions that facilitate genetic reassortment or direct transfer of avian viruses to humans. However, new viruses with pandemic potential could also arise elsewhere. In fact, human–avian reassortant viruses have been found in Italy and the Netherlands. Also, the 2003 H7N7 fowl plague outbreak in the Netherlands, with a fatal human infection (see below), underlines the risk of reassortment or adaptation in humans, and indicates that new viruses with pandemic potential need not necessarily arise in China. Alternatively, an old pandemic human virus (e.g. the H2N2 subtype) could be reintroduced from a hidden reservoir anywhere in the world.

It is not possible to predict when the next pandemic will strike. Since 1889, pandemics have occurred at intervals ranging from 10 to 40 years. A cyclic theory has been proposed suggesting that pandemics may appear in a specific recurring pattern.[25] The interval between the 1889 (H2) and 1900 pandemics (H3) matches that between the 1957 (H2) and 1968 (H3) pandemics. However, the approximate 20-year interval between the 1900 and 1918 pandemics would have predicted a global outbreak around 1988, 20 years after the 1968 pandemic, but this did not occur.

It is also important to re-emphasize that the emergence of a new virus subtype alone is not sufficient for a new pandemic to develop. Therefore, the occasional recent transmissions of H5N1 virus to humans, while underscoring that the threat is very real, do not by themselves herald a new pandemic. Additional changes of the virus are required, including the ability of the virus to spread among humans.

"Near misses" of the recent past

"H5N1" (1997–2004)

It is widely assumed that the mass slaughter of 1.5 million chickens in December 1997 in the Hong Kong H5N1 outbreak may well have averted a potential new human pandemic. Since this incident, the H5N1 virus has re-emerged several times. There is evidence that the precursor viruses of the H5N1 bird flu virus, including the goose H5N1 virus, remained in circulation.[27] Since 1998, culling has also included geese to prevent the goose H5N1 precursor virus from taking a firm hold in poultry in Hong Kong.

In May 2001, and in February and April 2002, the H5N1 virus was once again detected in Hong Kong's poultry markets.[7,28] It had apparently crossed from geese to ducks, undergone reassortment and then crossed to other poultry, but caused no human infections. However, in February 2003, a 9-year-old boy was hospitalized with an influenza A H5N1 illness, which also affected other members of his family. He survived but his father and 8-year-old sister died. Finally, in the spring of 2004, there was a major outbreak of highly pathogenic H5N1 avian influenza first detected in southern Vietnam and spreading quickly to neighbouring countries. To date (summer 2004 with the outbreak among poultry being under control), there have been 34 confirmed cases of human infection, 23 of whom died.[29,30] This underscores the extremely high pathogenicity of the H5N1 virus involved, which differed significantly from the 1997 H5N1 bird flu virus.

"H9N2" (1999)

In southern China, nine cases of human infection with an H9N2 avian virus were reported in 1998. In March 1999, there were two further cases in Hong Kong.[31] In no case was there serological evidence for H9N2 infection among family members or health care workers in close contact with the infected individuals, indicating that there was no human-to-human transmission. The virus was similar to one of the putative precursor viruses of the 1997 outbreak in Hong Kong. It appears that the H9N2 viruses are also circulating in pigs, together with human and porcine H1N1 and H3N2 viruses, providing conditions required for the generation of a reassortant virus with pandemic potential in humans.

"H7N7" (2003)

In the Netherlands in 2003, an outbreak of H7N7 fowl plague affected mainly poultry workers and veterinarians, causing conjunctivitis in most cases and an influenza-like illness in about 10%.[32] There was one death – a 57-year-old veterinarian who visited one of the infected farms and later died of acute respiratory distress syndrome. Mass culling of affected poultry was instigated and agricultural workers in contact with affected poultry were treated prophylactically with antiviral drugs. Also, these poultry workers were vaccinated for the human influenza strains circulating at the time to minimize dual infections as an opportunity for genetic reassortment.

Influenza surveillance and pandemic preparedness

The antigenic drift of influenza virus necessitates regular updates of the vaccine composition to optimise the match between the vaccine-induced antibodies and the anticipated virus (see pp. 124-151). To achieve as good a match as possible, in 1947, the WHO established an international Influenza Surveillance Network of laboratories to monitor the emergence and spread of new influenza strains around the world. This activity is coordinated by the WHO Collaborating Centres based in Atlanta, London, Melbourne and Tokyo. The work of the surveillance network has contributed greatly to our understanding of influenza epidemiology. It has also served and will continue to serve as a basis for an informed selection of strains for the next yearly influenza vaccine and the early detection of strains that could potentially cause a new influenza pandemic.

Notwithstanding the achievements of the WHO Influenza Surveillance Network, after the 1997 H5N1 outbreak in Hong Kong there is a growing recognition that more needs to be done. In response to this increasing awareness, the WHO has sought to raise the profile of influenza as a disease with a major public health impact throughout the world.[33] In 2002, the WHO adopted the Global Agenda on Influenza Surveillance and Control, which sets out a series of activities around four primary objectives: (i) strengthening surveillance, (ii) improving knowledge of disease burden, (iii) increasing vaccine usage, and (iv) accelerating pandemic preparedness. It is anticipated that the activities under the Global Agenda will facilitate an early detection of unusual influenza activity.

The Global Agenda will also contribute to an increased vaccination coverage in interpandemic periods[35] and to more efficient pandemic planning at the national level along the guidelines laid out in the WHO Influenza Pandemic Preparedness Plan.[36] Hopefully, an early detection of new influenza viruses with pandemic potential along with a swift institution of appropriate measures may allow us to avert a pandemic before it starts, or at least lessen its impact.

References

1. Wright PF, Webster RG. Orthomyxoviruses. In: Knipe DM, Howley PM, Griffin DE *et al.*, editors. Fields *Virology*, 4th edn. Lippincott Williams & Wilkins, 2001; pp. 1533–1579.

2. Rimmelzwaan GF, Boon AC, Voeten JT, Berkhoff EG, Fouchier RA, Osterhaus AD. Sequence variation in the influenza A virus nucleoprotein associated with escape from cytotoxic T lymphocytes. *Virus Res* 2004; **103**(1–2): 97–100.

3. Webster RG. 1918 Spanish influenza: the secrets remain elusive. *Proc Natl Acad Sci USA* 1999; **96**: 1164–1166.

4. Reid AH, Fanning TG, Hultin JV, Taubenberger JK. Origin and evolution of the 1918 "Spanish" influenza virus hemagglutinin gene. *Proc Natl Acad Sci USA* 1999; **96**: 1651–1656.

5. Gamblin SJ, Haire LF, Russell RJ *et al.* The structure and receptor binding properties of the 1918 influenza hemagglutinin. *Science* 2004; **303**: 1838–1842.

6. Webby RJ, Webster RG. Are we ready for pandemic influenza? *Science* 2003; **302**: 1519–1522.

7. Nicholson KG, Wood JM, Zambon M. Influenza. *Lancet* 2003; **362**: 1733–1745.

8. Webster RG, Laver WG. Determination of the number of nonoverlapping antigenic areas on Hong Kong (H3N2) influenza virus hemagglutinin with monoclonal antibodies and the selection of variants with potential epidemiological significance. *Virology* 1980; **104**:139–148.

9. Kilbourne ED. Influenza pandemics in perspective. *J Am Med Assoc* 1977; **237**: 1225–1228.

10. Fox JP, Cooney MK, Hall CE, Foy HM. Influenza virus infections in Seattle families, 1975–1979. II. Pattern of infection in invaded households and relation of age and prior antibody to occurrence of infection and related illness. *Am J Epidemiol* 1982; **116**: 228–242.

11. Webster RG. Influenza virus: transmission between species and relevance to emergence of the next human pandemic. *Arch Virol Suppl* 1997; **13**: 105–113.

12. Webster RG, Shortridge KF, Kawaoka Y. Influenza: interspecies transmission and emergence of new pandemics. *FEMS Immunol Med Microbiol* 1997; **18**: 275–279.

13. Horimoto T, Kawaoka Y. Pandemic threat posed by avian influenza A viruses. *Clin Microbiol Rev* 2001; **14**: 129–149.

14. Webster RG. Predictions for future human influenza pandemics. *J Infect Dis* 1997; **176**(Suppl 1): S14–S19.

15. Webster RG. Influenza: an emerging disease. *Emerg Infect Dis* 1998; **4**: 436.

16. Webster RG, Laver WG. Pandemic variation of influenza viruses. In: Kilbourne ED, editor. *The Influenza Viruses and Influenza*. Academic Press, 1975; pp. 269–314.

17. Webster RG, Bean WJ, Gorman OT, Chambers TM, Kawaoka Y. Evolution and ecology of influenza A viruses. *Microbiol Rev* 1992; **56**: 152–179.

18. De Jong JC, Claas ECJ, Osterhaus ADME, Webster RG, Lim WL. A pandemic warning? *Nature* 1997; **389**: 554.

19. Claas EC, Osterhaus AD, van Beek R *et al*. Human influenza A H5N1 virus related to a highly pathogenic avian influenza virus. *Lancet* 1998; **351**: 472–477.

20. Subbarao K, Klimov A, Katz J *et al*. Characterisation of an avian influenza A (H5N1) virus isolated from a child with a fatal respiratory disease. *Science* 1998; **279**: 393–396.

21. Nakajima K, Desselberger U, Palese P. Recent human influenza A (H1N1) viruses are closely related genetically to strains isolated in 1950. *Nature* 1978; **274**: 334–339.

22. Webster RG, Sharp GB, Claas EC. Interspecies transmission of influenza viruses. *Am J Respir Crit Care Med* 1995; **152**: S25–S30.

23. Bean WJ, Schell M, Katz J *et al*. Evolution of the H3 influenza virus hemagglutinin from human and nonhuman hosts. *J Virol* 1992; **66**: 1129–1138.

24. Guan Y, Shortridge KF, Krauss S, Webster RG. Molecular characterization of H9N2 influenza viruses: were they the donors of the "internal" genes of H5N1 viruses in Hong Kong? *Proc Natl Acad Sci USA* 1999; **96**: 9363–9367.

25. Potter CW. Chronicle of influenza pandemics. In: Nicholson KG, Webster RG, Hay AJ, editors. *Textbook of Influenza*. Oxford: Blackwell Science, 1998; pp. 3–18.

26. Beveridge WIB. The chronicle of influenza epidemics. *Hist Phil Life Sci* 1991; **13**: 223–235.

27. Guan Y, Shortridge KF, Krauss S *et al.* H9N2 influenza viruses possessing H5N1-like internal genomes continue to circulate in poultry in southeastern China. *J Virol* 2000; **74**: 9372–9380.

28. Guan Y, Peiris JSM, Lipatov AS *et al.* Emergence of multiple genotypes of H5N1 avian influenza viruses in Hong Kong SAR. *Proc Natl Acad Sci USA* 2002; **99**: 8950–8955.

29. Li KS, Guan Y, Wang J *et al.* Genesis of a highly pathogenic and potentially pandemic H5N1 influenza virus in eastern Asia. *Nature* 2004; **430**: 209–213.

30. Chen H, Deng G, Li Z *et al.* The evolution of H5N1 influenza viruses in ducks in southern China. *Proc Natl Acad Sci USA* 2004; **101**: 10452–10457.

31. Peiris M, Yuen KY, Leung CW *et al.* Human infection with influenza H9N2. *Lancet* 1999; **354**: 916–917.

32. Fouchier RA, Schneeberger PM, Rozendaal FW *et al.* Avian influenza A virus (H7N7) associated with human conjunctivitis and a fatal case of acute respiratory distress syndrome. *Proc Natl Acad Sci USA* 2004; **101**: 1356–1361.

33. Stöhr K. The global agenda on influenza surveillance and control. *Vaccine* 2003; **21**: 1774–1748.

34. World Health Organization. Influenza agenda on influenza. Adopted version Part I. *Wkly Epidemiol Rec* 2002; **77**: 179–182; Part II. *Wkly Epidemiol Rec* 2002; **77**: 191-196.

35. World Health Organization. Influenza vaccines. *Wkly Epidemiol Rec* 2000; **75**: 281–288.

36. World Health Organization. Influenza Pandemic Preparedness Plan. The role of WHO and guidelines for national or regional planning. 1999. http://www.who.int/csr/resources/publications/influenza/WHO_CDS_CSR_EDC_99_1/en/

The Immune Response to Influenza Infection

When the influenza virus infects the cells of the respiratory tract, both innate and adaptive immune responses are stimulated. Innate immune responses control virus replication during the early stages of infection, but require rapid activation of the adaptive immune response to prevent the infection from progressing to severe illness. The innate immune response recognizes virus-infected cells through mechanisms that are not antigen-specific, and restricts replication and spread of the virus during the early stages of infection. Cytokines produced by the innate immune response facilitate activation of antigen-specific adaptive immune mechanisms.[1] Binding of viral RNA to toll-like receptors (TLRs) on antigen-presenting cells (macrophages and dendritic cells)[2] and stimulation of immunological memory from prior exposure to viral antigens (natural exposure or through vaccination) also stimulates specific pathways in the adaptive immune response. Stimulation of the adaptive immune response by peptides derived from viral proteins ultimately leads to antibody production and activation of cytotoxic T lymphocytes (CTLs).[3] Figure 16 details many of the interactions of these different cell populations.

Antibodies bind to and neutralize the virus on the mucosal surface to prevent entry and replication inside the cell. These antibodies are largely strain-specific. Antigen-presenting cells determine how effectively T cells will be stimulated to produce antibodies and activate CTLs (see Figure 17). T helper (T_h1 and T_h2) cytokines reciprocally down-regulate each other and only T_h1 cytokines facilitate

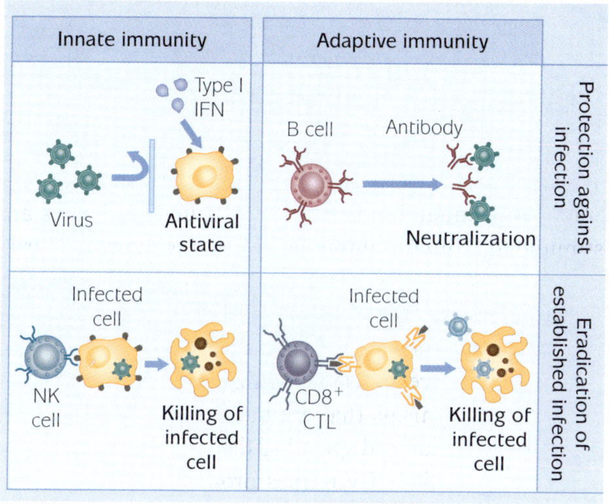

Figure 16. Immune responses to viral infections. Innate immune mechanisms include the production of cytokines and the activation of antigen-presenting cells (macrophages and dendritic cells) and natural killer (NK) cells. The adaptive, antigen-specific, immune response involves both the generation of antibodies by B cells and the activation of both T helper cells (mainly CD4-positive T cells) and CTLs (mainly CD8-positive T cells). Antibodies restrict the spread of virus primarily by neutralizing the virus so that it cannot enter the cell and replicate. CTLs recognize and destroy virus-infected cells, shortening the duration of viral shedding, and are responsible for clearing virus-infected cells from the lungs. Reproduced from Abbas AK, Lichtman AH. *Cellular and Molecular Immunology*, 5th edn. W.B. Saunders, 2003 with permission from Elsevier.

CTL activation.[4] Activation of CTLs and the associated increase in granzyme B (Grz B) that leads to programmed cell death (apoptosis) of virus-infected cells is likely to be

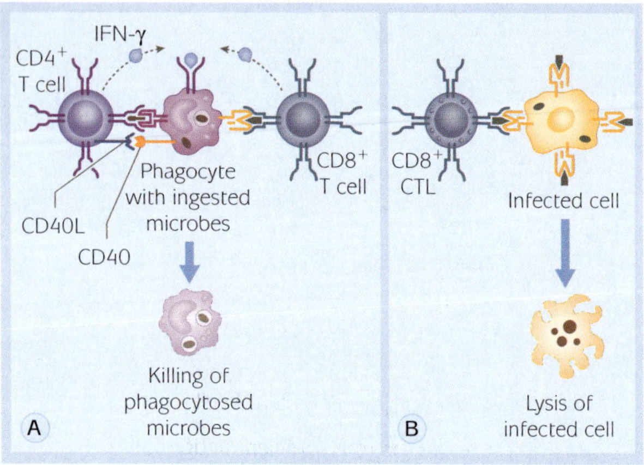

Figure 17. Cell-mediated immunity. **A.** The interaction of the CD4-positive ($CD4^+$) T cell with the antigen-presenting cell results in cytokine production. T_h1 (IFN-γ) cytokines stimulate antibody production and CTL activity and memory. **B.** Activated CTLs recognize viral peptide presented on the surface of an infected respiratory epithelial cell. This binding triggers apoptosis (programmed cell death) through a granule-mediated process to lyse the infected cell. If T_h2 cytokines are produced, CTLs are not activated. Adapted from Abbas AK, Lichtman AH, Pober JS. *Cellular and Molecular Immunology*. W.B. Saunders, 1999 with permission from Elsevier.

a critical component of antiviral immunity.[5] With ageing, antibody titres as a sole measure of protection against influenza become less reliable and the loss of CTL-mediated immunity has been directly linked to the increased risk of influenza illness in older people. This chapter will focus mainly on the adaptive immune response with reference to how this response may be altered by vaccination (reviewed in Ref. 6).

Key Messages

- Innate immune responses control influenza virus replication during the early stages of infection.
- Adaptive immune responses are antigen-specific and develop immunological memory that provides a more rapid response upon re-exposure to the virus.
- Secretory antibodies prevent infection at mucosal surfaces of the respiratory tract. Circulating antibodies diffuse to and protect the lungs.
- Cytotoxic T lymphocytes (CTLs) contribute to elimination of the infection by lysing virus-infected cells.
- Dendritic cells are the most efficient antigen-presenting cells, stimulating T cells.
- T helper type 1 (T_h1) responses stimulate antibody production (IgG2a) and CTLs. T helper type 2 (T_h2) responses stimulate antibody production (IgG1), but not CTLs.
- Immunological memory for B-cell responses is lifelong, and subtype- and strain-specific. In contrast, T-cell memory is more cross-reactive among different subtypes of influenza, while the duration of T-cell memory is variable, even among younger adults (months to years).
- Since antibodies are strain-specific, influenza vaccine composition must be updated regularly for protection against newly circulating strains of the virus.
- A significant decline in CTL-mediated immunity is directly linked to the increased risk of influenza illness in older people.

The innate immune response

Key features of the innate response

The "innate immune response" is stimulated when cells are infected with a virus. The influenza virus induces chemokine and cytokine production by infected epithelial cells and monocytes/macrophages. These chemokines attract immune cells to the site of infection, including macrophages, neutrophils and natural killer (NK) cells, as summarized in Table 5. These in turn produce additional cytokines, chemokines and other antiviral proteins.[7] This process activates a number of immune cells, including those of the adaptive immune response.

Interferons (IFN-α/β) are among the most important cytokines produced by the innate immune response and have several important antiviral functions as follows:

- They bind to neighbouring cells and induce an antiviral state by promoting the production of several intracellular antiviral proteins that inhibit protein synthesis (including, of course, viral proteins).
- They recruit monocytes/macrophages and T cells (including NK cells).

Components of the innate immune response	
	Innate system
Cellular components	Monocytes/macrophages
	Neutrophils
	Eosinophils
	Basophils
	Mast cells
	Natural killer cells
Secreted components	Complement
	Cytokines
	Lysozyme
	Acute phase proteins
	Interferons

Table 5. Components of the innate immune response. Reproduced from Griffin J *et al. Crash Course: Immunology and Haematology*, 2001 with permission from Elsevier.

- They stimulate increased major histocompatibility complex (MHC) class I and II molecule expression, resulting in enhanced antigen presentation, which facilitates adaptive immune mechanisms.
- They enhance maturation of antigen-presenting cells (APCs), to increase antigen presentation and stimulation of the adaptive immune response.

Virus infection of epithelial cells in the airways and lungs leads to presentation of viral peptides on MHC I. NK cells are large granular lymphocytes that detect virus-infected cells due to alterations in MHC I. During the early phase of infection, NK cells are activated through binding to MHC I–viral peptide complex and induce apoptotic cell death by releasing the contents of their granules into the infected cell.[8] The innate immune response is activated within a few hours of infection and lasts for 1–2 days.

Implications for the immunopathogenesis of influenza

High levels of cytokines are produced in the inflammatory, antiviral response to the large quantities of virus that may be produced in the absence of an adaptive immune response. Desquamation of the respiratory epithelium combined with inflammatory processes leads to transudation of large amounts of fluid into the lungs. Progressive hypoxia and acute respiratory distress syndrome may cause death within the first 1–2 days of the onset of illness. This process is more likely to occur with pandemic influenza where an unvaccinated individual has not had prior exposure to the subtype of influenza and must rely on the innate immune response to decrease viral replication. The adaptive immune system must mount a primary response, which is delayed because of lack of prior exposure to the subtype of influenza virus.

The adaptive immune response

Interferons, macrophages and NK cells slow virus replication and prevent the spread of virus during the first few days of infection. However, as is seen in individuals whose immune systems are naive to the infecting strain of virus, such as in infants or with pandemic strains of influenza, the innate immune response may not be enough to stem the spread of viral infection. Thus, survival relies on the "adaptive immune response" that is initiated during this period and is essential to eliminate the virus completely. This involves the activation of antigen-specific B and T lymphocytes and the production of antibodies. In individuals with previous exposure to the same antigen, the adaptive immune response is activated much more quickly due to "immunological memory".

The key feature of the adaptive immune response is the ability to store "immunological memory" for a specific pathogen. This memory provides a more rapid adaptive immune response that is specifically targeted to the antigens contained in that pathogen. Immunological memory results from genetic alterations within virus-specific B and T cells that become programmed to respond to a specific epitope, in this case of the viral antigens. Vaccination targets the adaptive immune response to stimulate circulating antibodies and an army of virus-specific T cells that are activated upon re-exposure to the pathogen during natural infection.

Structure and function of MHC

The adaptive immune response is activated when T cells recognize viral peptides presented by the major histocompatibility complex (MHC). The T helper cells produce cytokines that, along with direct antigenic stimulation of B cells and CTLs, lead to antibody production and CTL-mediated killing respectively. The MHC is a cluster of tightly linked genes, found on the short arm of chromosome 6. Gene products of the MHC are involved in peptide binding, processing and presentation. MHC molecules allow the immune system to distinguish "self" from "non-self" and to detect the presence of pathogens. T cells recognize antigens in the context of MHC molecules.

MHC genes exhibit a high degree of polymorphism. This means that individuals exhibit unique MHC and the diversity of the MHC increases the likelihood that a protective adaptive immune response can be mounted by most people. Class I and class II MHC molecules are glycoproteins expressed on the cell surface, and consist of cytoplasmic, transmembrane and extracellular portions. The specificity of MHC is largely concentrated in the peptide-binding cleft, but the overall structure of MHC enables the immune system to distinguish self from non-self. T cells are only able to recognize viral antigens presented by self-MHC molecules (self-MHC restriction). CD8-positive T cells recognize antigen only in association with class I MHC molecules (MHC I restricted), while CD4-positive T cells recognize antigen only in association with class II MHC molecules (MHC II restricted).

Antigen processing and presentation

MHC molecules present peptide fragments derived from viral proteins either degraded or synthesized inside the cell, and the MHC–peptide complex is transported to the cell surface, where the complex can be recognized by the T-cell receptor. Antigen-presenting cells have different pathways of antigen processing for class I and class II MHC, and different requirements for loading peptides from live or killed virus on the MHC I (see Figure 18). In contrast to other APCs, including macrophages, dendritic cells are able to present peptides derived from any form of virus, including killed viruses, through what have been defined as "non-classical" pathways. The ability of dendritic cells to deliver viral protein antigens from the endosomal compartment to the cell cytosol for processing in the MHC class I pathway is important in the context of the development of new inactivated influenza vaccines that will induce not only an adequate antibody response but also CTL activity, as discussed on pages 166–189.

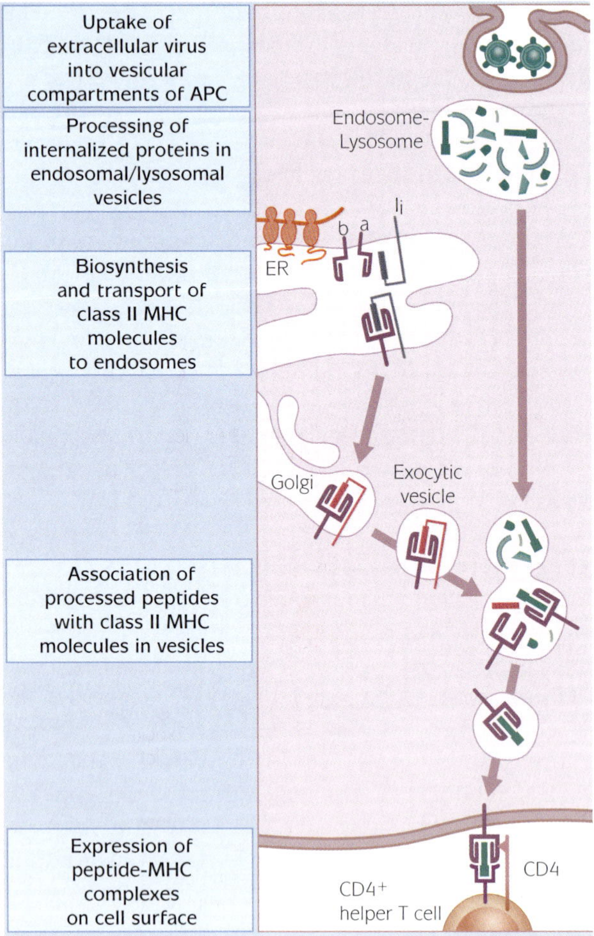

Figure 18. Pathways of antigen processing and presentation. Peptides presented on class II MHC are processed from antigens taken up by endocytosis by the antigen-presenting cell and loaded onto MHC II for presentation to the CD4-positive (CD4$^+$; helper) T cell. Peptides presented on class I MHC are derived from cytosolic proteins taken up by proteosomes, the peptides incorporated during synthesis of the MHC I molecule and

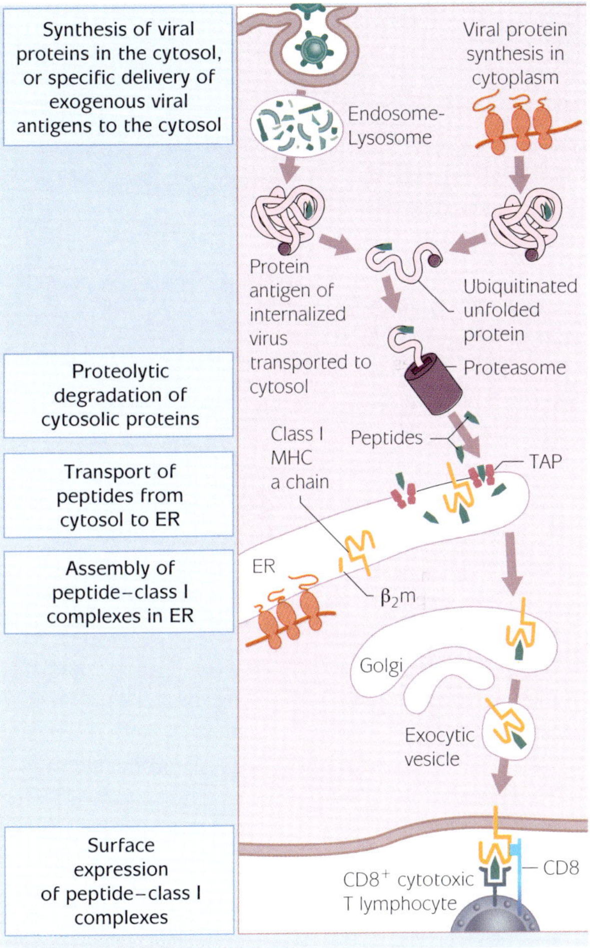

presented to the CD8-positive (CD8+; cytotoxic) T cell. Antigen-presenting cells present viral peptides derived from replicating virus inside the cell. Dendritic cells also have the unique capability of being able to present peptides derived from exogenous virus taken up by the cell. Adapted from Abbas AK, Lichtman AH. *Basic Immunology*, 2nd edn. W.B. Saunders, 2004 with permission from Elsevier.

Professional APCs process and present antigen to T helper cells (CD4-positive T cells) in association with MHC II, and to CTLs (CD8-positive T cells) in association with MHC I. APCs express high levels of MHC II and variable amounts of MHC I depending on the degree of up-regulation of MHC I by interferon-gamma (IFN-γ). Professional APCs include:

- Dendritic cells – the key APC due to the presence of both classical and non-classical pathways for antigen presentation on MHC I.
- Macrophages.
- B cells.

CD4 and CD8 are “accessory” molecules that play an important role in the T-cell–antigen interaction (see Figure 18). CD4 and CD8 have two important functions:

- They bind MHC class II and class I molecules respectively, thereby strengthening the T-cell–antigen interaction.
- They function as signal transducers.

Antibodies to HA neutralize the virus

Influenza virus stimulates an adaptive immune response in both bone marrow-derived lymphocytes (B cells) and thymus-derived lymphocytes (T cells), resulting in humoral and cell-mediated immunity respectively. Studies of the response to vaccination in adults and children over the age of 4 years old typically represent restimulation of a previously primed response through exposure to natural infection or prior vaccination. Virus-activated T cells, through a variety of cytokine mediators, stimulate B cells to differentiate and produce antibodies that are specific for the strains of virus contained in the vaccine. These specific antibodies bind to the surface glycoproteins, haemagglutinin (HA), as shown in Figure 19, and neuraminidase (NA). As a result, anti-HA antibodies block attachment and cell entry of the virus particles, thus effectively neutralizing the virus. NK cells also bind to antibody–virus complexes on the surface of virus-infected cells and kill by antibody-

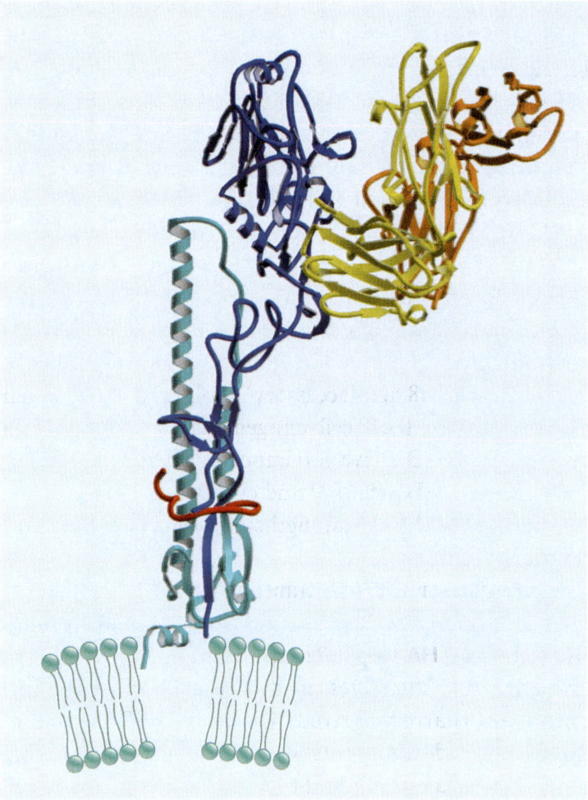

Figure 19. Mechanism of influenza virus neutralization by an antibody directed against the viral HA. The figure shows the three-dimensional structure of an HA monomer (in blue), with (in yellow) an attached Fab (antigen-binding) fragment of an antibody specific for epitope D of HA (see Figure 7). This figure was produced, using MOLSCRIPT, on the basis of the co-ordinate file from the Protein Data Bank, code 1EO8. Fleury D *et al*. Structural evidence for recognition of a single epitope by two distinct antibodies. *Proteins Struct Funct Genet* 2000; **40**: 572.

dependent cell-mediated cytotoxicity (ADCC) as part of the adaptive immune response.

The peptide sequences on the outer surfaces of HA and NA change as a result of selective pressure by the immune system against the native virus, a phenomenon known as antigenic drift (see pp. 45–67). Mutant viruses thus produced may escape antibody binding due to changes in the antigenic determinants of the B-cell response. Influenza vaccines are updated annually to ensure that immunity is stimulated to the relevant predicted strains of the H3N2 and H1N1 subtypes of influenza A and influenza B (see pp. 124–151). Increased attack rates when vaccine strains are mismatched with the circulating strains of influenza are well documented. Even with a good match between the vaccine and circulating strain of virus, B-cell activation and antibody production are not enough to control influenza virus infection. In addition, infected cells need to be cleared from the system in order to prevent the formation of new virus particles. This is achieved by the activation of T cells.

CTLs are critical for clearance of influenza virus and recovery from illness

The importance of CTLs in clearing virus from infected lung tissue has been clearly demonstrated. Human studies showed that CTL activity is important for recovery from influenza infection even in the absence of protective antibodies to the infecting virus strain.[9] CTLs combat influenza viral infections by recognizing and destroying virus-infected host cells that become the factories for viral replication. Infected cells expressing on their surfaces the MHC I–viral peptide complex are recognized by and activate virus-specific CTLs. The mechanisms by which CTL activation leads to lysis of virus-infected cells include perforin- or granule-mediated killing.[3] Granule-mediated killing appears to be the critical effector function of CTLs against influenza infection.

Virus-specific, granule-mediated killing results from the production of granules within CTLs that contain pore-forming proteins (perforins) and granzymes (Figure 20). Granules are transported to the surface of activated CTLs at the point of contact with an appropriate target cell. Through a process facilitated by perforin, granzymes are

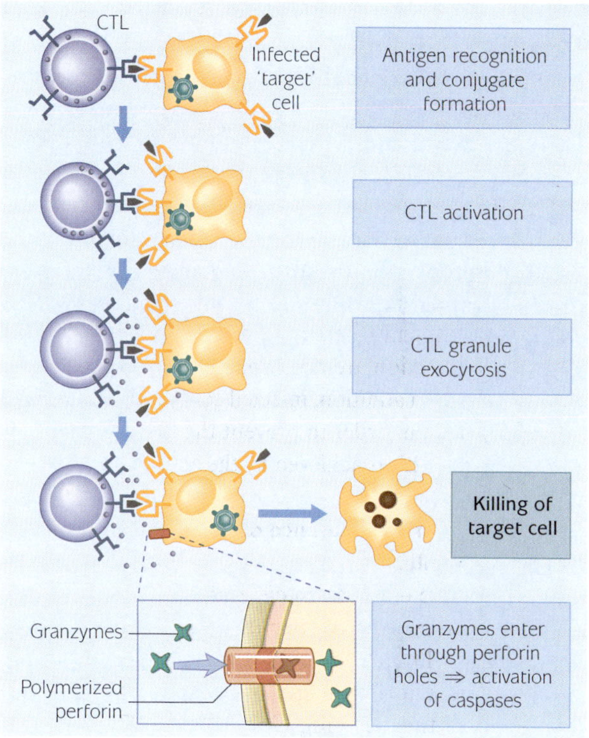

Figure 20. Mechanism of CTL-mediated killing. Granules in the CTL migrate to the cell surface upon CTL activation and cross into the virus-infected cell to induce apoptotic cell death through DNA fragmentation and disruption of mitochondrial metabolism. Reproduced from Abbas AK, Lichtman AH. *Basic Immunology*, 2nd edn. W.B. Saunders, 2004 with permission from Elsevier.

transported across the cell membrane into the cytoplasm of the target cell and are involved in an enzymatic cascade that eventually results in DNA fragmentation and cell death (apoptosis). The combined activity of Grz B and perforin is important for target-cell lysis. Thus, the activation of CTLs and associated increase in Grz B that leads to apoptotic cell death is likely to be a critical component of antiviral immunity.

Importance of T-cell responses in adaptive immunity

T-cell responses are conserved across different strains of influenza

There are two main cell types within the T-lymphocyte population, helper T cells (T_h) and cytotoxic T lymphocytes (CTLs). In contrast to B cells, which have a subtype- and strain-specific response, the antigenic determinants of the T-cell response are more conserved across the different strains of influenza.[10] Internal peptide sequences of HA and NA are similar within the subtypes of influenza (e.g. A/H3N2 vs. A/H1N1) and the internal viral proteins (matrix and nucleoproteins (NP)) are conserved within the types of influenza (e.g. influenza A vs. influenza B). The T_h response is stimulated by peptides derived from the surface glycoproteins that are conserved within the subtypes of influenza A (H3N2 and H1N1) or strains of influenza B. The internal proteins also stimulate T_h as well as CTL responses. These responses are much more cross-reactive compared to antibody responses, but recent data suggest that antigenic drift also affects CTL responses against NP as soon as immunological pressure is applied.[11] That means that the expected cross-reactivity of CTL responses across all strains may not be the case. The immunological memory for B-cell responses is lifelong, and subtype and strain specific. In contrast, T-cell memory is much more cross-reactive within the different types of influenza, and estimates of the duration of T-cell memory after priming with influenza are highly variable, from months to years, even among younger adults.[2]

Helper T-cell responses to influenza are important for CTL memory

Helper T cells recognize antigens presented by MHC II; MHC II is expressed almost exclusively on APCs, B cells and T cells. In contrast, CTLs recognize viral peptides in combination with MHC I; MHC I is expressed on most cells in the body. Because of the different requirements for antigen presentation on MHC I and MHC II, T_h and CTL activations are independently determined by the form of the viral antigen, and the interaction with a specific MHC, its cellular location and the specific APC type. The fact that vaccines containing inactivated virus can stimulate CTLs in primed populations suggests an interaction between dendritic cell non-classical pathways for antigen presentation on MHC I and restimulation of T-cell memory. New technologies in vaccine or vaccine adjuvant development may be helpful for enhancing this interaction and stimulating a more robust CTL response to influenza vaccination.

Implications of a T_h1 versus T_h2 response to influenza vaccination

The T_h-mediated immune response to influenza virus plays a key role in the generation of both humoral and CTL-mediated responses to influenza vaccination. Subsets of T_h cells are defined by the cytokines that they produce when stimulated.[7,12] Naive T_h cells (no prior exposure to antigen) produce mainly interleukin-2 (IL-2). Memory T_h cells, when restimulated, produce cytokine profiles of the T_h1 or T_h2 type. T_h1 cytokines include IL-2 and IFN-α; T_h2 cytokines include IL-4, IL-5 and IL-10. Since IL-10 suppresses T_h1 cytokine production and IFN-α suppresses T_h2 cytokines, the cytokine response represents either a T_h1 or T_h2 response to vaccination. T_h1 responses stimulate both antibody production and CTLs, while T_h2 responses stimulate antibody and not CTL production. Thus, a T_h1 or T_h2 response can stimulate antibody production while only T_h1 stimulates a CTL response. Thus, the measurement of antibody titres as a correlate of the T-cell response does not necessarily distinguish between a T_h1 and a T_h2 response, and how effectively CTL memory is restimulated by vaccination.

Effect of ageing on the immune system

Ageing leads to a decline in cell-mediated immunity relative to humoral immune mechanisms. There may be a loss with ageing in the quality of antibodies produced, but the increased risk of influenza illness more closely parallels the changes in T-cell function. Ageing is associated with decreased production in IL-2 (T_h1) and a related loss of the T-cell proliferative response to antigenic stimulation, increased IL-4 (T_h2) production and a decline in CTL responses, suggesting a general shift toward the less protective T_h2 cytokine response to influenza and diminished protection against influenza illness. Vaccination may stimulate T_h1 cytokines and CTL memory, but these responses are less robust even in healthy older people compared to younger adults, and may be further compromised by chronic diseases and associated functional decline.

CTL responses to influenza decline with advancing age and frailty

Ageing is associated with a decline in CTL activity, related responses to vaccination and a delay in recovery from illness. Current inactivated influenza vaccines stimulate a CTL response in older and even chronically ill adults, although CTL activity in general is lower in older compared to young adults and is not as robust as the response to natural infection. A significant decline in CTL-mediated immunity and related Grz B production is directly linked to the increased risk of influenza illness in older people.[13]

References

1. Durbin JE, Fernandez-Sesma A, Lee CK *et al.* Type I IFN modulates innate and specific antiviral immunity. *J Immunol* 2000; **164**: 4220–4228.

2. Diebold SS, Kaisho T, Hemmi H *et al.* Innate antiviral responses by means of TLR7-mediated recognition of single-stranded RNA. *Science* 2004; **303**: 1529–1531.

3. Doherty PC, Topham DJ, Tripp RA *et al.* Effector CD4+ and CD8+ T-cell mechanisms in the control of respiratory virus infections. *Immunol Rev* 1997; **159**: 105–117.

4. Doherty PC, Allan W, Eichelberger M, Carding SR. Roles of alpha beta and gamma delta T cell subsets in viral immunity. *Ann Rev Immunol* 1992; **10**: 123–151.

5. Johnson BJ, Costelloe EO, Fitzpatrick DR *et al*. Single-cell perforin and granzyme expression reveals the anatomical localization of effector CD8+ T cells in influenza virus-infected mice. *Proc Natl Acad Sci USA* 2003; **100**: 2657–2662.

6. Esser MT, Marchese RD, Kierstead LS *et al*. Memory T cells and vaccines. *Vaccine* 2003; **21**: 419–430.

7. Julkunen I, Melen K, Nyqvist M, Pirhonen J, Sareneva T, Matikainen S. Inflammatory responses in influenza A virus infection. *Vaccine* 2000; **19**(Suppl 1): S32–S37.

8. Trapani JA, Smyth MJ. Killing by cytotoxic T cells and natural killer cells: multiple granule serine proteases as initiators of DNA fragmentation. *Immunol Cell Biol* 1993; **71**(Pt 3): 201–208.

9. McMichael AJ, Gotch FM, Noble GR, Beare PA. Cytotoxic T-cell immunity to influenza. *New Engl J Med* 1983; **309**: 13–17.

10. Effros RB, Doherty PC, Gerhard W, Bennink J. Generation of both cross-reactive and virus-specific T-cell populations after immunization with serologically distinct influenza A viruses. *J Exp Med* 1977; **145**: 557–568.

11. Rimmelzwaan GF, Boon AC, Voeten JT *et al*. Sequence variation in the influenza A virus nucleoprotein associated with escape from cytotoxic T lymphocytes. *Virus Res* 2004; **103**: 97–100.

12. Mosmann TR, Cherwinski H, Bond MW *et al.* Two types of murine helper T cell clone. I. Definition according to profiles of lymphokine activities and secreted proteins. *J Immunol* 1986; **136**: 2348–2357.

13. McElhaney JE, Gravenstein S, Upshaw CM *et al*. Granzyme B: a marker of risk for influenza in institutionalized older adults. *Vaccine* 2001; **19**: 3744–3751.

Pathogenesis, Clinical Features and Diagnosis

The rapid evolution of both influenza A and B viruses is the major cause of the occurrence of annual flu epidemics in people. Influenza A is particularly important due to the threat of pandemic strains that may arise from avian reservoirs of this virus subtype, as discussed on pages 45–67.

Generally, flu is a self-limiting respiratory infection. The influenza virus does not normally spread beyond the respiratory tract, primarily because the protease required for cleavage of the viral HA is restricted to the epithelium of the airways and lungs (see pp. 23–44). As a result, the virus is rarely found circulating in the blood or in other organs. Host factors such as interferons and other components of the immune response may also be important for preventing the spread of the virus outside of the respiratory tract. When a new influenza A subtype is introduced into the human population, the situation may be different. The severity of disease may be considerably increased because of the complete lack of immunity in infected individuals under these conditions. Additional alterations in viral proteins may have contributed to the extremely high pathogenicity of the H1N1 pandemic strain of 1918 and that of the more recent avian H5N1 virus, which infected several tens of people with a very high case-fatality rate.[1]

Influenza is a common illness during the winter months, but the overlap of symptoms with other respiratory illnesses and the practitioner's knowledge of whether influenza is circulating in the community is key to the diagnosis. The severity of illness depends on the age of the patient (the very old and the very young are most susceptible to serious illness), whether or not high-risk conditions (chronic heart, lung and kidney diseases, diabetes or immunosuppressive conditions) are present, and whether or not the person has been vaccinated. Thus, physician knowledge about influenza in the community combined with an understanding of the individual risk of complications of influenza is required for clinical decision-making with respect to vaccination and antiviral drugs for prevention or treatment of influenza.[2]

Key Messages

- The rapid evolution of influenza A and B viruses contributes to annual flu epidemics. Only influenza A causes pandemics due to its ability to undergo genetic reassortment.
- Physician awareness is the single most important factor in the diagnostic accuracy of influenza. It is essential therefore that primary-care physicians be well informed about local influenza surveillance data (see Appendix 1).
- Proper and rapid diagnosis is essential to control influenza infections by antiviral treatment and to avoid the inappropriate use of antibiotics.
- Influenza spreads by aerosols or droplets – it can persist in the air and on hands or fomites for significant periods of time.
- The pathogenesis of influenza is based on mucosal inflammation and lysis of respiratory epithelial cells.
- Influenza virus does not normally spread beyond the respiratory tract due to the limited tissue distribution of proteases involved in activation of HA.
- Systemic symptoms of influenza are mainly due to circulation of the inflammatory cytokines produced in response to infection.
- Age, co-morbid illness and vaccination status affect the presentation of illness and are key determinants of illness severity.
- Considering that older people may lose up to 2–3% of muscle power per day of bed rest, significant disability may result from influenza illness.
- Pandemic influenza and the recent experience with H5N1 strains demonstrate the potential threat of influenza in unprimed populations.

Pathogenesis of influenza

Beyond the virus-related properties that determine pathogenesis, the different types of influenza are of variable clinical importance in people. The influenza A H3N2 subtype is usually associated with greater mortality than the H1N1 subtype and the influenza B virus. Influenza C causes clinically unimportant illness. The effects of influenza on the naive immune system are evident in the high-risk population of children under the age of 2 years, with some protection mediated by maternal antibodies in infants less that 6 months old.[3] Elderly people are particularly at risk for influenza illness, because of ageing effects on the immune system and the greater incidence of underlying medical conditions. The more co-morbid the conditions, the greater the risk. People in residential care are particularly susceptible because they are generally older, have a high rate of chronic ill health, live in close proximity to each other (facilitating transmission) and respond less well to vaccination. Interestingly, the current cohort of older people appears to be less susceptible compared to young adults and children when H1N1 strains circulate in the community.[4] This protection of older adults against H1N1-mediated illness has been attributed to priming with H1N1 strains that circulated during their childhood and generated protective immunologic memory.

Mode of transmission

The primary mode of transmission is by aerosol or droplets. The virus may remain suspended in the air for long periods of time and can be dispersed by air currents. Transmission may also occur by contact with virus-contaminated hands or fomites. Inhaled virus may be trapped in mucus produced by airway epithelial cells and then transported by the cilia to the posterior pharynx, where it is swallowed or expectorated ("tracheal toilet"). This mechanism may be impaired in chronic obstructive lung disease, asthma or debilitated people.

Lysis of respiratory epithelial cells

The influenza virus causes a lytic infection of respiratory epithelial cells (see pp. 23–44). As a consequence, mucosal cells become vacuolated, oedematous and desquamate, leaving only the basal cells and the basement membrane of the respiratory epithelium. The resulting exudative process with increased mucus production causes a runny nose, cough and nasal congestion. In uncomplicated influenza, acute diffuse mucosal inflammation and oedema of the upper airway and bronchi are observed. In older people, cough is the most common presenting feature of influenza illness, often in the absence of other more classic symptoms such as fever and myalgias, but these symptoms do not distinguish influenza from other viral respiratory illnesses.[5]

With viral pneumonia, there is an interstitial pneumonitis with a predominantly mononuclear leucocyte infiltration. The alveolar walls become denuded of epithelium; hyaline membranes form, and the intra-alveolar space becomes filled with exudate and haemorrhage from the surrounding capillaries, significantly impairing diffusion of gases. Progressive hypoxia occurs as the alveolar space is obliterated. In pandemic influenza, where the immune system has no immunological memory for the infecting virus strain, this may be a common scenario even in healthy young people.[2]

Immunopathogenesis

The immune response to influenza has been presented in the previous chapter. This section discusses the immunopathogenesis of influenza – how the body's response to the virus contributes to the symptoms of influenza. Inflammatory cytokines, including tumour necrosis factor-alpha (TNF-α) and alpha- and beta-interferons (IFN-α, IFN-β), have been associated with the pathogenesis of influenza infection. Although critical components in the down-regulation of intracellular protein synthesis to limit new virus production, these cytokines, along with interleukins (IL-1β, IL-6) produced by the adaptive immune response, are largely responsible for the systemic symptoms of influenza illness, including fever and myalgias. Importantly, influenza virus is limited to the lungs except in rare circumstances where infections of muscles and the central nervous system have been documented. Local symptoms such as cough and sore throat may be a combination of desquamation of the epithelial lining of the airways and the resulting inflammatory response to necrosis of the cells in the process of viral replication. In particular, plasma IL-6 levels correspond to the severity of respiratory symptoms and fever in community-acquired influenza A illness, although serum levels of a number of other cytokines are elevated as well.[6] Paradoxically, older people often do not mount a fever with influenza infection, even though IL-6 levels increase with age. In children, influenza-mediated upper respiratory illness is an important cause of acute otitis media, but the association with cytokine levels has not been determined.[7]

Pathogenesis of pandemic influenza

The increased severity of illness with pandemic influenza (see pp. 45–67) relates primarily to the profound inflammatory response that is stimulated in immunologically naive individuals to suppress viral replication while the adaptive immune response is activated. Destruction of respiratory epithelium from viral replication and the inflammatory exudates produced may lead to profound hypoxia and death within hours to 2–3 days of the onset of illness, as illustrated in the text box opposite, describing the typical disease picture caused by the Spanish flu virus. In spite of extensive RNA sequence analyses of the 1918 virus, other properties contributing to its extreme pathogenicity are still not completely understood.[8,9]

As shown in Figure 21, death was age related during interpandemic years, with high mortality rates in the under 5-year-olds and the very elderly. During influenza pandemics, the mortality curves were W-shaped, reflecting the higher attack rates that are generally seen in healthy

"There was clear evidence of ... shortage of breath and the appearance of mahogany spots around the mouth which would extend and coalesce into a violaceous heliotrope cyanosis until 'a white man could not be distinguished from a coloured'. A peculiar stench emanated from many patients. With increasing cyanosis, patients begin to gasp for breath; blood-stained fluid would froth from the mouth; patients would become delirious, and death would follow from suffocation. With rigor mortis, bloody fluid would gush from the mouth and nostrils. The time from hospital admission to death could be a few hours to 2–3 days."

***Textbook of Influenza* (Ref. 30)**

young adults (25–49 years old) but with higher mortality rate in this population compared to interpandemic years. The highest incidence was in 5- to 14-year-olds, but they had the lowest mortality. Death was frequently due to primary viral pneumonia (usually uncommon) or secondary bacterial pneumonia (antibiotic treatment was not yet available).

Attack rates of Asian flu (1957–58) varied in different communities around the world. Groups with the highest infection rates included schoolchildren aged 5–14 years (>50%), the institutionalized and those living in crowded conditions. Overall, mortality was only 10% of that seen with the Spanish flu, but despite this, it translated into 33,000 excess deaths during the second wave in the UK, and 39,000 and 20,000 excess deaths during the first and second waves respectively in the USA. Many factors have been postulated to explain differences in attack rates, but these have yet to be determined (reviewed in Ref. 2).

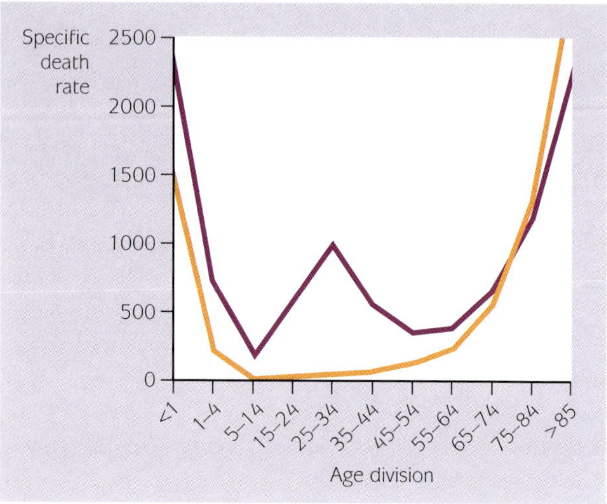

Figure 21. Influenza and pneumonia mortality by age in the USA. Influenza- and pneumonia-specific mortality by age, including the pandemic year 1918 and the average of the interpandemic years 1911–15, is shown. Specific death rate is per 100,000 of the population for each age division. Purple line, 1918 pandemic; orange line, average of interpandemic years 1911–15. Adapted from Potter CW, editor. *Influenza (Perspectives in Medical Virology)*, 2003 with permission from Elsevier.

Presentation of uncomplicated influenza

The clinical presentation of influenza ranges from an asymptomatic infection or a self-limiting upper respiratory tract infection (URTI) to a severe illness, often with serious, potentially fatal, complications.[10] The incubation period is 1–4 days, with an average of 2 days. The clinical course is dependent on the virulence of the virus. The age of the patient (the very young and the old), and the presence of chronic medical illness (such as cardiac and pulmonary diseases), immunosuppression and pregnancy increase the severity of illness.

The typical uncomplicated influenza A syndrome is a symptom complex that overlaps with a number of other respiratory illnesses. There is an abrupt onset, with high-grade fever (38–40°C) being the most prominent symptom. Other symptoms include headache, chills, dry cough, myalgias, malaise and anorexia. In more extreme cases, severe malaise with prostration is observed. Respiratory symptoms such as rhinorrhoea, nasal congestion and sore throat are present, but are overshadowed by the systemic symptoms during the first 3 days of illness. The influenza virus tends to remain in the respiratory tract and does not usually cause a viraemia. Systemic symptoms are due to proinflammatory cytokines, which are released following activation of the host's defence mechanisms (see pp. 68–85). The cough frequently changes from a dry, hacking nature to one that is productive of small amounts of sputum that are usually mucoid but can be purulent. After the fever and upper respiratory tract symptoms resolve (usually within 7–10 days), cough and weakness can persist for 1–2 additional weeks. The frequency of influenza symptoms in adults, shown in Figure 22, may vary with the age of the patient, as discussed below.

Effect of age on clinical presentation

Influenza attack rates are higher in children compared to adults. High-grade fever, cervical lymphadenopathy, and nausea and vomiting are frequent manifestations of influenza in children. Drowsiness (uncommon in adults) occurs in about 50% of under fours, and in up to 10% of 5- to 14-year-olds. Otitis media is frequently present (25% overall), particularly in those prone to middle ear infections (67% in 1- to 3-year-olds). In infants (under 5 years old), 5–10 per thousand are hospitalized with respiratory symptoms (acute bronchitis, croup, pneumonia), and one in 5000 dies during influenza epidemics.

Elderly patients experience more lower respiratory tract symptoms, with productive cough, wheeze and chest pain. In older adults, cough is the most common presenting

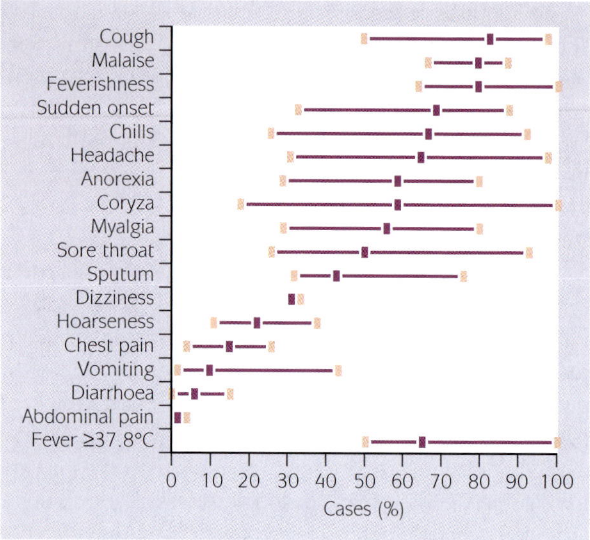

Figure 22. Influenza symptoms and their associated frequencies. Data are from 10 studies involving 520 adults with uncomplicated influenza A. Adapted from Nicholson KG. Human influenza. In: Nicholson KG, Webster RG, Hay AJ, editors. *Textbook of Influenza*. Oxford: Blackwell Science, 1998; pp. 219–264 with permission from Blackwell Publishing.

symptom (in greater than 80% of cases), while fever is much less common compared to young adults. Considering that older people may lose up to 2–3% of muscle power per day of bed rest, significant disability may result from influenza illness. It is therefore not surprising that influenza and pneumonia represent one of the six leading causes of catastrophic disability in the age 65 and older populations.[11] Gastrointestinal symptoms also tend to be more common, especially with influenza B. Between four and 10 elderly patients per thousand are hospitalized. Vaccination has been associated with a drop in this admission rate by 39% overall, and with a drop of 27% in admissions for heart failure, suggesting that many of them are influenza related, and underscoring the frequency of cardiovascular complications in the elderly. In addition, vaccination has been associated with reduction in cardiovascular events (32% for myocardial infarction and 20% for strokes).[12] These observations point to the inflammatory basis of influenza illness and related complications.

Complications of influenza

Influenza-associated pneumonia

In otherwise healthy individuals, influenza infection normally results in an uncomplicated URTI that resolves within 1–2 weeks. However, pneumonia is a relatively common complication (5–38% with influenza A and 10% with influenza B), predominantly in the elderly, patients with chronic cardiopulmonary disease, pregnant women and immunocompromised individuals. The aetiology may be viral, bacterial or mixed viral–bacterial.[10] Such patients can deteriorate rapidly and mortality can be close to 50%.[13]

In primary viral pneumonia, typical influenza is followed by a rapid progression (over 2–3 days) of fever, cough, dyspnoea, chest pain and cyanosis. Physical examination and chest X-ray disclose diffuse bilateral infiltrates consistent with adult respiratory distress syndrome. If fatal, death usually occurs within 4–5 days of first symptoms.

Combined viral–bacterial pneumonia is more common than primary viral pneumonia. Of patients with a severe pneumonia, 75% will have secondary bacterial infection. In these cases, the individual will appear to be recovering from the influenza illness and then have a recurrence of the respiratory symptoms. The bacteria most commonly involved are *Staphylococcus aureus* and *Streptococcus pneumoniae*, with *Haemophilus influenzae* being less common. There is evidence that influenza infection actively facilitates the pathogenicity of bacteria and the impact of illness, causing immunosuppression. In the 1957–58 pandemic, mortality from staphylococcal pneumonia (28%) was similar in all age groups and twice as high as mortality from other pneumonias (12%), which tended to occur in the elderly and those with chronic medical conditions. Once the responsible pathogen has been identified, appropriate antibiotic treatment should be initiated promptly.

Bacterial pneumonia as a complication of influenza has a different presentation from primary viral pneumonia. In this case, patients initially show clinical improvement from an influenza illness and then develop worsening respiratory symptoms. In this case, physical and chest X-ray examinations are more likely to show localized signs of consolidation.

Influenza B virus can cause the same spectrum of disease as that seen after influenza A virus infection, and severe illness can occur, particularly in the elderly.

Other respiratory complications

Exacerbations of asthma, chronic obstructive pulmonary disease and cystic fibrosis are common complications of influenza illness. Acute bronchitis develops in 30% of cases and, less commonly, lung abscess and empyema may be observed. Three-quarters of children with asthma will suffer an exacerbation. In hospitalized children, influenza accounts for 16% of asthmatic exacerbations and 4–13% of exacerbations of cystic fibrosis. The most common respiratory complications in hospitalized children are acute bronchitis (12–26%), croup (5–15%) and pneumonia (5–8%).

Non-respiratory complications

Myositis is reported more frequently in children with influenza B, but adults may also be affected and may develop rhabdomyolysis with acute renal failure.[14] Cardiac complications, specifically myocarditis, have been described in patients with influenza A and B, but these complications are mostly asymptomatic.[15] Pericarditis has been reported rarely. ECG abnormalities are common and usually transient (81% of hospitalized patients, 43% of community patients), but underlying conditions can cause fatal arrhythmias or cardiomyopathies. CNS complications are rare and range from irritability and confusion to psychosis and severe encephalopathy due to a variety of inflammatory processes, including Reye's syndrome.[16] Recovery is usually complete.

The link between the 1918–20 pandemic and encephalitis lethargica remains unproven. Guillain–Barré syndrome has been reported after influenza vaccination.[17] Febrile convulsions are common in hospitalized children (20–50%).[18]

Influenza in susceptible subgroups

Table 6 summarizes the high-risk populations for significant morbidity and mortality from influenza. These groups should be targeted for vaccination and other means of prophylaxis, as well as optimal disease management. Additional prophylaxis strategies include encouraging vaccination of close contacts of these individuals. These include family members and other household or institutional contacts.

People at high risk of hospitalization or death from influenza
People in specific age categories • adults aged 65 years and older • children under age 2 years
People with chronic disease • chronic pulmonary disease (asthma, bronchitis, emphysema, tuberculosis) • chronic cardiovascular disease • diabetes mellitus • renal disease
Immunocompromised people • transplant recipients • HIV-positive people • splenic dysfunction
Pregnant women

Table 6. People at high risk of hospitalization or death from influenza. Adapted from World Health Organization. Influenza vaccines. *Wkly Epidemiol Rec* 2000;**75**:281–288.

Older adults and adults with chronic diseases

As discussed above, influenza poses increased risks to the elderly (>65 years old), who have a higher incidence of chronic medical conditions. In these patients, influenza may occur as a serious illness, with exacerbation of underlying conditions and possibly fatal outcome (reviewed in Ref. 19). Cough is the most common presenting symptom of influenza in this population and presents a diagnostic challenge to the physician.[20] More than 90% of influenza-associated excess deaths occur in the age 65 and older population, and thus prevention, diagnosis and appropriate management of illness significantly impact health outcomes in this population.[21] People aged 50–65 years are also at greater risk due to the increased rate of chronic medical conditions, such as diabetes and cardiac, pulmonary or renal diseases, and immunocompromising conditions or medications. All of these conditions are associated with a significant increase in risk of hospitalization and death, and also require optimal disease management along with vaccination for the prevention of influenza illness.

Children

Infants and children under the age of 2 years will generally have a naive immune system and potentially compromised ability to mount an effective immune response to influenza. Morbidity and mortality are highest in this paediatric population. Additional common risk factors are related to asthma and type 1 diabetes, as well as immunocompromising conditions, although these are less common. School absentee rates can exceed 50% during influenza epidemics and provide evidence of the highly contagious nature of this illness. The diagnostic accuracy of influenza in children and the relationship to diagnostic testing has been recently reviewed.[22]

Immunocompromised patients

Influenza is more common in immunocompromised individuals (32%) than community controls (14%) and can cause severe disease.[23] Pneumonia (usually viral) is more common and mortality is higher. In a study of adults with leukaemia and adult recipients of haematopoietic stem cell transplants, severe lymphopenia, elderly age, receipt of an allogeneic haematopoietic stem cell transplant and concurrent opportunistic infections were identified as independent risk factors for a complicated course. Prolonged shedding of influenza virus (up to 5 months) and rapid emergence of resistance to amantadine and rimantadine have been observed in immunocompromised individuals.[24] HIV infection does not appear to be associated with more severe illness.

Pregnant women

Women in the second or third trimester of pregnancy have an increased risk of hospitalization due to cardiorespiratory complications.[25] The risk is greatest in pregnant women with mitral valve disease, who have a 45% mortality rate associated with influenza infection (higher if labour occurs during influenza infection).

Diagnosis of influenza

The accuracy of diagnosis of influenza tends to be strongly dependent on the physician's awareness of whether or not there is influenza activity in the local community. In clinical trials, accuracy of diagnosis during epidemics reached 62%, but may be as reliable as near-patient rapid testing (see below) when influenza is known to be circulating in the local community. Given the non-specific clinical presentation, the accuracy of diagnosis during epidemics is quite good. However, outside epidemic periods diagnostic accuracy may be less than 10%. Thus, it is important that primary-care physicians be aware of local influenza surveillance data (see list of websites in Appendix 1).

The differential diagnosis of an influenza-like illness (ILI) includes a variety of viruses (e.g. respiratory syncytial virus, parainfluenza virus, rhino- and coronaviruses, and adenoviruses) and bacteria (e.g. mycoplasma, chlamydia, rickettsia).

Proper and rapid diagnosis is essential to control influenza infection by antiviral treatment and to avoid the inappropriate use of antibiotics – the latter is a perennial problem, particularly in southern European countries. Accurate diagnosis is also very important for selection of vaccine virus strains and for the purposes of influenza surveillance.

Table 7 lists the criteria for the clinical diagnosis of influenza that have been used in trials of antiviral drugs. Additional criteria are used in epidemiological studies to estimate attack rates and vaccine effectiveness, and apply clinical case definitions during the peak influenza period.[26] The most specific clinical case definition of influenza is "febrile upper respiratory illness" (URI), defined as 2 days of URI symptoms (runny nose, sore throat, cough) with two or more symptoms on at least 1 day and fever on at least 1 day.

A case definition of intermediate sensitivity and specificity is "any URI", defined as 2 days of at least one URI symptom (runny nose, sore throat, cough). The most

Criteria for clinical diagnosis of influenza
Fever (≥ 37.8°C) and/or feverishness
plus
TWO of: • Cough • Sore throat • Nasal symptoms • Myalgia • Headache • Malaise

Table 7. Criteria for clinical diagnosis of influenza. Reproduced from Nicholson KG. *Managing Influenza in Primary Care*, 1999 with permission from Blackwell Publishing.

sensitive clinical case definition of influenza is "any URI symptom", defined as any 1 day with at least one symptom (fever, runny nose, sore throat, cough, headache, muscle aches, chills, tiredness/weakness). The specificity of these case definitions is highly dependent on the attack rates of influenza in the community.

Thus, as indicated above, up-to-date tracking and awareness of circulating influenza in the local community is the single most important factor in the diagnostic accuracy of identifying influenza as a cause for an acute respiratory tract illness.

Diagnostic tests

Diagnostic tests available for influenza include virus isolation and culture, antigen or viral RNA detection, and serology. However, the sensitivity and specificity vary widely, and the positive and negative predictive value of these tests is highly dependent on whether or not influenza is circulating in the local community – the contribution of these tests to clinical diagnosis thus needs to be carefully considered.[27] Rapid influenza tests have been developed but have some limitations (see below under "Antigen detection"). Appropriate samples for influenza testing include nasopharyngeal or throat swabs, nasal wash or nasal aspirates, depending on which type of test is used. Samples should be collected within the first 4 days of illness. Acute and convalescent serum samples can be tested for influenza antibodies. Viral culture or reverse transcriptase–polymerase chain reaction (PCR) remains essential for determining the influenza subtypes and strains causing illness.

Serology

Influenza viruses cause agglutination of erythrocytes due to the capacity of the viral HA to bind to sialic acid residues on the red blood cell surface (see pp. 23–44). Anti-HA antibodies interfere with this process and the haemagglutination–inhibition (HI) test is based on these properties (see pp. 124–151). A four-fold or greater increase in HI antibodies is indicative of infection (this occurs in about 70–90% of cases). Sera must be pre-treated to prevent false-positive results. The HI assay is used routinely to assess the response to vaccination.

Virus isolation and culture

The influenza virus can be isolated from cell culture or from chicken embryos. In the latter, they produce haemagglutinating activity, the entire process taking about 4–5 days, although more rapid (less sensitive) methods are available. Because influenza may not produce cytopathic effects in cell culture, the haemagglutinating unit is used to screen for evidence of viral replication.

Antigen detection

Antigen can be detected by a variety of immunological techniques, including direct immunofluorescence of respiratory secretions, indirect antibody staining of exfoliated nasal epithelium or commercially available rapid influenza diagnostic tests. The latter differ in their ability to detect and distinguish between influenza A and B virus infections, methodologies, processing time and cost. The sensitivities of the rapid tests are lower than viral culture of respiratory specimens and may be comparable to symptom-defined illness when influenza is known to be circulating in the local community; a negative result might not exclude influenza virus infection. Rapid influenza tests provide results within 24 hours, while viral culture takes 3–10 days.

RNA detection by PCR

Although labour-intensive and usually slower than other tests, reverse transcriptase–PCR is used to type and subtype influenza infections.[28] Either clinical or cell culture specimens can be used. Multiplex PCR can differentiate between influenza A and B, parainfluenza 1, 2 and 3, and respiratory syncytial virus (RSV) with a very high degree of specificity (98%) and sensitivity (100%).

Influenza diagnosis in primary care

The diagnosis of influenza can be a particular challenge in the absence of surveillance data. Thus, the recommended approach for the patient who presents with an acute respiratory illness is to first determine whether or not a viral aetiology is likely according to symptom criteria, and whether or not influenza is circulating in the local community. During an influenza outbreak, the primary-care physician can make the diagnosis of influenza based on clinical diagnostic criteria with similar diagnostic accuracy to that provided by the current rapid diagnostic tests. However, these tests may be helpful in the early stage of an influenza outbreak to identify sentinel cases. In addition, the collection of patient samples for virus culture and identification is critical to maintaining the network for influenza surveillance that determines the onset, peak and resolution of an influenza activity in the community.[29] The primary mode of influenza prevention is vaccination (see pp. 124–151). Antiviral drugs provide additional prophylaxis, particularly in high-risk patients for whom influenza vaccination is contraindicated, and effective use of these drugs in the treatment of influenza (discussed on pp. 152–165) depends on the physician's confidence in the diagnosis of influenza.[30]

References

1. Guan Y, Poon LL, Cheung CY *et al.* H5N1 influenza: a protean pandemic threat. *Proc Natl Acad Sci USA* 2004; **101**: 8156–8161.

2. Nicholson KG, Wood JM, Zambon M. Influenza. *Lancet* 2003; **362**: 1733–1745.

3. Glezen WP, Taber LH, Frank AL, Gruber WC, Piedra PA. Influenza virus infections in infants. *Pediatr Infect Dis J* 1997; **16**: 1065–1068.

4. McBean AM, Hebert PL. New estimates of influenza-related pneumonia and influenza hospitalizations among the elderly. *Int J Infect Dis* 2004; **8**: 227–235.

5. Loeb M, McGeer A, McArthur M, Peeling RW, Petric M, Simor AE. Surveillance for outbreaks of respiratory tract infections in nursing homes. *Can Med Assoc J* 2000; **162**: 1133–1137.

6. Kaiser L, Fritz RS, Straus SE, Gubareva L, Hayden FG. Symptom pathogenesis during acute influenza: interleukin-6 and other cytokine responses. *J Med Virol* 2001; **64**: 262–268.

7. Vesa S, Kleemola M, Blomqvist S, Takala A, Kilpi T, Hovi T. Epidemiology of documented viral respiratory infections and acute otitis media in a cohort of children followed from two to twenty-four months of age. *Pediatr Infect Dis J* 2001; **20**: 574–581.

8. Reid AH, Taubenberger JK. The 1918 flu and other influenza pandemics: "over there" and back again. *Lab Invest* 1999; **79**: 95–101.

9. Webster RG. 1918 Spanish influenza: the secrets remain elusive. *Proc Natl Acad Sci USA* 1999; **96**: 1164–1166.

10. Cate TR. Clinical manifestations and consequences of influenza. *Am J Med* 1987; **82**: 15–19.

11. Ferrucci L, Guralnik JM, Pahor M, Corti MC, Havlik RJ. Hospital diagnoses, Medicare charges, and nursing home admissions in the year when older persons become severely disabled [see comments]. *J Am Med Assoc* 1997; **277**: 728–734.

12. Nichol KL, Nordin J, Mullooly J, Lask R, Fillbrandt K, Iwane M. Influenza vaccination and reduction in hospitalizations for cardiac disease and stroke among the elderly. *New Engl J Med* 2003; **348**: 1322–1332.

13. Ison MG, Hayden FG. Viral infections in immunocompromised patients: what's new with respiratory viruses? *Curr Opin Infect Dis* 2002; **15**: 355–367.

14. Berry L, Braude S. Influenza A infection with rhabdomyolysis and acute renal failure – a potentially fatal complication. *Postgrad Med J* 1991; **67**: 389–390.

15. Miura M, Asaumi Y, Wada Y *et al.* A case of influenza subtype A virus-induced fulminant myocarditis: an experience of percutaneous cardio-pulmonary support (PCPS) treatment and immunohistochemical analysis. *Tohoku J Exp Med* 2001; **195**: 11–19.

16. Kimura S, Ohtuki N, Nezu A, Tanaka M, Takeshita S. Clinical and radiological variability of influenza-related encephalopathy or encephalitis. *Acta Paediatr Jpn* 1998; **40**: 264–270.

17. Lasky T, Terracciano GJ, Magder L *et al.* The Guillain–Barré syndrome and the 1992–1993 and 1993–1994 influenza vaccines [see comments]. *New Engl J Med* 1998; **339**: 1797–1802.

18. Heininger U. An update on the prevention of influenza in children and adolescents. *Eur J Pediatr* 2003; **162**: 828–836.

19. Loeb M. Pneumonia in the elderly. *Curr Opin Infect Dis* 2004; **17**: 127–130.

20. Widdicombe J, Kamath S. Acute cough in the elderly: aetiology, diagnosis and therapy. *Drugs Aging* 2004; **21**: 243–258.

21. Janssens JP, Krause KH. Pneumonia in the very old. *Lancet Infect Dis* 2004; **4**: 112–124.

22. Uyeki TM. Influenza diagnosis and treatment in children: a review of studies on clinically useful tests and antiviral treatment for influenza. *Pediatr Infect Dis J* 2003; **22**: 164–177.

23. Vilchez RA, Fung J, Kusne S. The pathogenesis and management of influenza virus infection in organ transplant recipients. *Transpl Infect Dis* 2002; **4**: 177–182.

24. Englund JA, Champlin RE, Wyde PR *et al.* Common emergence of amantadine- and rimantadine-resistant influenza A viruses in symptomatic immunocompromised adults. *Clin Infect Dis* 1998; **26**: 1418–1424.

25. Lim WS, Macfarlane JT, Colthorpe CL. Treatment of community-acquired lower respiratory tract infections during pregnancy. *Am J Respir Med* 2003; **2**: 221–233.

26. Nichol KL, Mendelman P. Influence of clinical case definitions with differing levels of sensitivity and specificity on estimates of the relative and absolute health benefits of influenza vaccination among healthy working adults and implications for economic analyses. *Virus Res* 2004; **103**: 3–8.

27. File TM. Community-acquired pneumonia. *Lancet* 2003; **362**: 1991–2001.

28. Templeton KE, Scheltinga SA, Beersma MF, Kroes AC, Claas EC. Rapid and sensitive method using multiplex real-time PCR for diagnosis of infections by influenza A and influenza B viruses, respiratory syncytial virus, and parainfluenza viruses 1, 2, 3, and 4. *J Clin Microbiol* 2004; **42**: 1564–1569.

29. Meerhoff TJ, Meijer A, Paget WJ. Methods for sentinel virological surveillance of influenza in Europe – an 18-country survey. *Eur Surveill* 2004; **9**: 1–4.

30. Potter CW. Chronicle of influenza pandemics. In: Nicholson KG, Webster RG, Hay AJ, editors. *Text-book of Influenza*. Oxford: Blackwell Science, 1998.

Social and Economic Impact of Influenza

The societal burden of recurring annual influenza epidemics and, in particular, occasional pandemics is often underestimated. It is important to understand the extent to which influenza impacts on society, its financial burden and strategies to minimize the impact. This chapter provides an overview of the social and economic implications of influenza. It introduces economic concepts and methods, and examines the impact of influenza on different population groups (including children, working adults and the elderly) and sectors of the economy (health care and workplace).

Each outbreak of influenza takes a significant toll on societies in terms of morbidity, mortality and financial resources.[1,2] For example, the WHO estimates that there are 3–5 million cases of severe influenza illness, resulting in 250,000–500,000 deaths annually in the industrialized world. Vaccination is the most important strategy for preventing influenza. Yet, data on vaccination coverage as discussed in the next chapter show that even in industrialized countries, large proportions of the population at risk do not receive the influenza vaccine. The target of the WHO of reaching 75% vaccination coverage of high-risk people therefore remains an important goal for 2010. Achieving this target will also have major positive implications for the capacity of individual countries to respond adequately to influenza pandemics. The chapter finishes with a brief look at the social and economic impact of influenza pandemics. The health benefits as well as the cost-effectiveness of influenza vaccination will be discussed in the next chapter.

Key Messages

- The WHO estimates that 3–5 million cases of severe influenza illness result in 250,000–500,000 deaths annually in the industrialized world.
- Compared to healthy adults, influenza-related death rates are as much as 50- to 100-fold higher among patients with cardiovascular or pulmonary disease, and even higher for those with two or more co-morbid conditions.
- In young children, influenza is associated with increased rates of otitis media and serious cardiorespiratory illnesses leading to hospitalization.
- The annual cost of influenza is highly variable and may be as high as €20 million in direct health care costs in some European countries – these direct costs are less than 10% of the total annual cost to society.
- Work absenteeism from influenza illness results in indirect costs that may also be as high as $20 million in lost days of work in a single influenza season.
- School absenteeism not only impacts on children but contributes on average to a loss of 3 work days for the parent who must remain at home with the child.
- Intangible costs include those related to death, increased disability or a diminished quality of life for the individual and the potential additional burden to caregivers.
- The Centers for Disease Control (CDC) has estimated that in the USA, during an influenza pandemic, high-risk individuals representing 15% of the population would account for ~84% of all deaths, at a cost of US $71.3–166.5 billion, excluding disruptions to commerce and society.

Social impact

In addition to the short-term incapacitating symptoms of influenza, complications directly and indirectly arise from having influenza. These complications have a large social impact, including increased demands on health care systems, long-term illness and disability, and even mortality.

Epidemiological records on the morbidity and mortality statistics related to influenza show that, in the winters from 1990 to 1998, the mean annual estimate of influenza-associated deaths in the USA was 51,203, mostly associated with influenza A (H3N2).[3] The death rates varied from year to year, with an average across the decade of 19.49 influenza-related deaths per 100,000 population (Table 8).

The influenza attack rate varies from year to year, as does the virus strain. The annual influenza attack rate lies between 6000 and 12,000 per 100,000 population. In addition to excess deaths, influenza also results in extra hospitalizations that range from 70 to 160 per 100,000

Estimated annual influenza deaths rates per 100,000 in the USA (1990–1999)

Season	A/H1N1	A/H3N2	B	Total
1990–1991	0.79	2.41	7.00	10.20
1991–1992	2.57	18.11	0.22	20.90
1992–1993	0.46	7.75	7.42	15.64
1993–1994	0.07	18.88	0.16	19.10
1994–1995	0.22	12.91	2.72	15.85
1995–1996	5.58	8.94	2.84	17.36
1996–1997	0.00	20.98	4.73	25.71
1997–1998	0.02	26.27	0.24	26.54
1998–1999	0.11	20.39	3.57	24.07
Mean	**1.09**	**15.18**	**3.21**	**19.49**

Table 8. Estimated annual influenza deaths rates per 100,000 in the USA (1990–1999). Reproduced from Thompson WW *et al.* Mortality associated with influenza and respiratory syncytial virus in the United States. *JAMA*; **289**: 179–186[3] with permission from the American Medical Association. US Population Estimates Program at www.census.gov/.[4]

Estimated annual morbidity and excess mortality in Europe during a moderate influenza epidemic

Country	Inhabitants (millions)	Influenza-like illness (millions)	Excess hospitalizations (thousands)	Excess deaths
Austria	8	0.48–0.96	5.6–12.8	400–1200
Belgium	10	0.6–1.2	7.0–16.0	500–1500
France	56	3.36–6.72	39.2–89.6	2800–8400
Germany	77	4.62–9.24	53.9–123.2	3850–11,550
Italy	55	3.3–6.6	38.5–88.0	2750–8250
Portugal	10	0.6–1.2	7.0–16.0	500–1500
Spain	40	2.4–4.8	28.0–64.0	2000–6000
Switzerland	7	0.42–0.84	4.9–11.2	350–1050
The Netherlands	15	0.9–1.8	10.5–24.0	750–2250
UK	56	3.36–6.72	39.2–89.6	2800–8400

Table 9. Estimated annual morbidity and excess mortality in a number of European countries during a moderate influenza epidemic. Data taken in part from Palache AM. *Influenza vaccination: The effect of dose and age on the antibody response. A methodological evaluation of serological vaccination studies*, 1991. PhD thesis, Erasmus University Rotterdam, the Netherlands.

population. Table 9 shows estimated ranges of influenza-like illness cases, and associated hospitalizations and deaths for the USA and for a number of European countries.

Population groups at higher risk

As discussed in the last chapter, complications arising from influenza are more frequent and serious among adults with chronic conditions, such as pneumonia and respiratory disease, cardiac disease and cerebrovascular disease.[5] Influenza may cause secondary bacterial pneumonia and exacerbations of underlying chronic medical conditions that can result in hospitalization and even death. These groups are at a higher morbidity and mortality risk from influenza.

Death rates associated with influenza and pneumonia have been estimated as two per 100,000 for patients with no high-risk conditions, 10 per 100,000 in those with one high-risk condition and 377 per 100,000 in those with two or more high-risk conditions.[6] Other studies have reported that influenza-related death rates are as high as 50 times greater in patients with cardiovascular disease, 100 times greater in patients with pulmonary disease, and even higher in those with two or more co-morbid conditions, than in healthy adults.[7] Indeed, fatalities from influenza rise from around 45 years of age and are highest among people with chronic medical conditions.

Typically, the elderly are more at risk from chronic conditions and therefore it is observed that death rates from influenza are higher among the elderly, where up to 90% of influenza-related deaths are observed. However, it is still debated if age itself is an independent risk factor.

Among children, the largest high-risk group are those with asthma, which accounts for approximately 7% of children. These children have considerably more outpatient visits, antibiotic courses and higher hospitalization rates during all seasons than other children at increased risk.[8] In young children, influenza may be associated with increased rates of otitis media and even more serious cardiorespiratory illnesses leading to hospitalization (Table 10).

Influenza-related health care interventions among children	
	Excess number per 1000 children
Hospitalizations for children:	
• <1 year of age	19
• 1 to ≤ 3 years of age	8
• Outpatient visits	200
• Courses of antibiotic therapy	140

Table 10. Influenza-related health care interventions among children. Reproduced from Neuzil KM *et al*. The burden of influenza illness in children with asthma and other chronic medical conditions. *J Pediatr* 2000; **137**: 856–864[8] with permission from Elsevier.

Economic impact

In addition to the social impact of influenza, with increased morbidity and mortality , influenza also has a significant economic impact, including lost and reduced workplace and social productivity due to incapacitating symptoms, and increased health care costs from treating the symptoms.

Understanding the economics of influenza

The economics of influenza are concerned primarily with two issues: the economic impact of influenza and the cost of interventions to prevent or treat influenza. The economic impact of disease is often measured by conducting a cost of illness study, which estimates the overall cost of the disease, including its treatment and consequences. These costs can be classified into three separate types:

- Direct costs – these are actually incurred monetary costs, and imply a cash outlay (acquisition costs, fees, charges).

- Indirect costs – these are not paid in cash but can be inferred, as they arise from reduced or lost productivity due to work absenteeism, decreased performance or even premature death.
- Intangible costs – these are attributable to pain, suffering and reduced quality of life. Avoidance of these is often identified as an intangible benefit. These costs cannot be easily converted to a monetary value.

In influenza, the cost of prevention or treatment strategies, such as influenza vaccination programmes, may be measured using cost-effectiveness analyses or cost-benefit analyses. These analyses of influenza-related health care interventions measure whether the benefits derived from the intervention are worth the cost of undertaking the intervention.

The costs of the intervention are typically measured from the perspective of the payer (e.g. health care system) and include the direct cost of the intervention itself. The benefits, on the other hand, can include direct, indirect and intangible costs resulting from the intervention. These may include reduced hospitalizations and physician visits, reduced work or school absenteeism, reduced mortality and improved quality of life. Reduced health care visits can provide a cost saving to the health care payer. Reduced absenteeism at work is an indirect benefit to the employer and society. Reduced mortality and improved quality of life is an intangible benefit that is gained by the individual, their family and friends, and society at large.

Economic evaluations estimating the cost-effectiveness of programmes should always compare one health care strategy against another. For example, when estimating the cost-effectiveness of influenza vaccination, the analysis may compare the expected overall cost and benefits of no vaccination against the expected costs and benefits resulting from an influenza vaccination programme. The decision-maker would then be presented with the additional costs of the vaccination programme and be asked if it is worth the additional cost given the additional benefits it provides during the influenza season.

The results from such analyses are usually presented in the form of an incremental cost-effectiveness ratio (ICER), which shows the additional cost of providing the vaccination programme per extra additional unit of benefit. This can be illustrated with a simple hypothetical example. Suppose a programme to vaccinate 1000 people costs $100,000. The vaccination reduces health care resource use, saving the health care payer $50,000. Furthermore, by reducing the number of people with influenza, the programme also avoids five deaths relating to influenza. Therefore, the ICER would be:

($100,000 – $50,000)/5 = $10,000 per life saved.

If the decision-maker would normally be prepared to pay more than $10,000 to save a life, the programme would be deemed a cost-effective option. If the programme can avoid more costs than it costs to implement, and it saves more lives, then the programme is always cost-effective as it provides more benefit and saves money.

A cost-benefit analysis converts all effectiveness benefits, including intangible costs, into a monetary value. In the example above, the decision-maker may value a life saved at $30,000. Consequently, the monetary benefit of the programme is $50,000 (health care savings) plus $150,000 (five lives saved at a value of $30,000 each). This total monetary benefit of $200,000 outweighs the $100,000 cost of implementing the programme. The programme would therefore be deemed cost-effective and should be implemented.

Cost of illness

The increasing cost of health care has prompted research to quantify the cost of illness due to influenza. Cost of illness research is the first step in resource allocation decision-making; it can increase awareness of the impact of infection, determine the burden of disease in relation to other diseases, define the unmet medical need which future drug development should address, and facilitate the formulation of prevention, vaccination and treatment policies. Such research is hampered by underestimates of the incidence of the disease and difficulties quantifying indirect and intangible costs. Studies in France and Germany have shown that the annual cost of influenza is US $20,346,000 and US $1,970,000, with between 8.3% and 8.7% of these costs related to direct medical costs (see Tables 11 and 12).[9,10]

Direct costs

The direct costs of influenza have been estimated in a number of different studies. These vary depending on the structure of the national health services. Physician visits act as the main cost driver. In the USA, influenza affects approximately 50–60 million people annually, of whom about 50% visit their doctor.[11] Most of these 25 million physician visits are by schoolchildren and young adults. Between 114,000 and 142,000 (2.1–2.6 per 1000) of those infected are hospitalized, mainly very young children (5 per 1000) and elderly people (3–4 per 1000).[12] The annual direct medical costs of influenza are estimated at between $3 and $5 billion.[13]

Reported studies of work loss due to influenza range from 0.79 to 4.9 days of work lost.[14] From a UK study, the mean time off work for health care workers was 4 days for those with influenza.[15] However, it has been noted that health care workers tend to continue to work during their illness.[16]

From the National Health Interview Survey in the USA, influenza was responsible for more than 200 million days of restricted activity, 100 million days of bed disability, 75 million days of lost work and 22 million health care provider visits in 1995.[14] Direct costs are higher for high-risk patients.

Indirect costs: work productivity loss and school absenteeism

The most significant cost of influenza to society is the indirect cost of lost productivity and absenteeism. Estimates of the cost of influenza in the USA, France and Germany have shown that indirect costs can be 5–10 times higher

Estimated cost of an influenza epidemic in France in 1989 (millions)

Costs	1989 (French francs)		2003 equivalent ($ US)	
	National health insurance system	Society	National health insurance system	Society
Direct medical costs:				
GP visits	363.95	494.20	516.99	702.01
medications	350.69	637.61	498.16	905.73
hospitalizations	92.39	115.49	131.24	164.05
Total direct medical costs	807.03	1247.31	1146.39	1771.81
Cost of absenteeism	1121.30	13076.00	1592.81	18574.52
Total costs	1928.33	14323.31	2739.20	20346.32

Table 11. Estimated cost of an influenza epidemic in France in 1989 (millions). Reproduced from Levy E. French economic evaluations of influenza and influenza vaccination. *Pharmacoeconomics* 1996; **9**(Suppl 3): 62–66[9] with permission from Adis International.

than direct costs and range from \$10 to \$15 billion per year. Such indirect productivity costs accounted for between US \$1,805,000 and US \$18,574,000 in Germany and France (see Tables 11 and 12, year 2003 prices).

Estimated cost of an influenza epidemic in Germany in millions (1996–97)			
	Costs		
Outpatient data observed	DM (1996–97)	\$ US (1996–97)	\$ US (2003)
Direct medical costs:			
consultation and examination	50.03	29.43	55.49
diagnostic	3.51	2.06	3.89
medication	23.25	13.6	25.79
Total medical direct costs	76.79	45.09	85.17
Indirect costs:			
loss of productivity	1591	936	1764.53
Total costs for outpatients	1668	981	1849.93
Inpatient data (modelled)			
Direct costs	72	42	79.85
Indirect costs	37	22	41.04
Total costs for inpatients	109	64	120.89
Overall total costs	1777	1045	1970.82

Table 12. Estimated cost of an influenza epidemic in Germany in millions (1996–97). Reproduced from Levy E. French economic evaluations of influenza and influenza vaccination. *Pharmacoeconomics* 1996; **9**(Suppl 3): 62–66[10] with permission from Adis International. Data derived from *Statistical Yearbook for Germany*, 1997.[10]

During influenza outbreaks, there is a significant rise in absenteeism in the working population. Surveillance programmes have found that the high absenteeism in the workplace is common during peak influenza activity, typically between December and March.[17] Overall, influenza accounts for around 10% of sickness absence from work.

Numerous studies have been conducted around the world estimating the effect of influenza-like illness (ILI) in the workplace. In the general population, it takes nearly 7 days on average to alleviate the major symptoms of ILI.[18] From a review of the literature, Nichol[14] concluded that workers with ILI took an average of 2 days off work. This was based on estimates in the literature ranging from 0.79 days[19] to 4.9 days.[20] Nichol *et al.*[21] estimated that for every 100 non-vaccinated employees, 52 working days were lost due to upper respiratory illness. Campbell and Rumley[22] estimated the direct costs of medical care received for ILI at $22.80 per person, and the indirect costs at $80 to the company for each day's absence from work. Other estimates for the cost per working day lost are higher; for example, in Dille,[17] where the cost per work day lost was estimated at $175.24.

Even a mild attack of influenza can reduce reaction times by 20–40%,[23] with associated health and safety implications in those who continue working despite influenza infection (up to half of employees). Workers who have ILI and either stay at work or return to work before the illness has disappeared have reduced effectiveness (lower productivity) while working. Keech *et al.*[24] calculated that workers, on average, returned to work 0.7 days before they should. As well as reduced effectiveness at work, there are additional burdens associated with making poor decisions when you are ill.

Burckel *et al.*[25] calculated mean attack rates for different levels of morbidity for various age groups based on information from Houston Surveillance and other European evidence, assuming an overall attack rate of 10%. The 18–24 age group was found to be most likely to contract low-morbidity influenza in which normal work schedules are essentially maintained and the related impairment was equivalent to an average of one lost day of work. In moderate influenza morbidity, 3 days of work were lost for patients under 45 years and 4 days for those over 45 years. High-morbidity influenza was defined as influenza cases that require hospitalization with an average of 12 days of work lost.[25]

In a study of families with school-aged children during the influenza season compared with the non-influenza winter season, there was a significantly greater total number of illness episodes, febrile illnesses, analgesic use, school absences, parental absenteeism and secondary illnesses among family members. It was concluded that the influenza season has significant adverse effects on the quality of life of school-aged children and their families.[26] Time off work due to children being away from school with influenza can also be an important factor. On average, 3 days of work are lost due to a child being absent from school because of influenza, requiring a parent to remain at home.[14]

Intangible costs

Intangible costs include quality of life and impairment of function and performance. Influenza infection is stressful for the individual infected and frequently places a burden of care on other family members. This can restrict the usual activities of families and reduce the quality of life of the affected individual, as well as those around him/her. The socio-economic impact of these factors is difficult to quantify. In elderly people, in particular, infection is associated with a decline in major physical functions.[27]

Impact of pandemic influenza

While the costs of epidemic influenza are considerable, the potential social and economic impact of pandemic influenza is even greater. It is always difficult to predict the impact of a future pandemic with a reasonably high degree of accuracy. Factors influencing the impact include the attack rate, the pathogenicity of the virus and the adequacy of control measures. Pandemic influenza results from the emergence and rapid spread of novel influenza viruses. The most devastating on record was the 1918–19 "Spanish flu" pandemic caused by an H1N1 virus, estimated to have caused between 20 million and 50 million deaths worldwide. Smaller pandemics, such as the 1957 Asian flu (A/H2N2) and the 1968 Hong Kong flu (A/H3N2), have caused less severe pandemics, but morbidity and mortality in the elderly and people with high-risk conditions remained severe.

The Centers for Disease Control has estimated the costs involved in the event of a pandemic in the USA.[28] Patients at high risk (15% of the population) would account for approximately 84% of all deaths, and the economic impact would be between US $71.3 and $166.5 billion, excluding disruptions to commerce and society (Table 13).

In the event of another pandemic, and particularly in light of rapid ageing of the population, a crisis in health care capacity and ability to cope may be anticipated along with a considerable social and economic impact.[29] One study using a 25% attack rate in the event of a pandemic estimated a 3.7-fold rise in outpatient visits, a 3.9-fold

Estimated socio-economic burden of a future influenza pandemic in the USA

Clinical event	Numbers affected
Deaths	89,000–207,000
Hospitalizations	314,000–734,000
Outpatient visits	18–42 million
Additional illnesses	20–47 million

Table 13. Estimated socio-economic burden of a future influenza pandemic in the USA. Data derived from Meltzer MI *et al*. The economic impact of pandemic influenza in the United States: priorities for intervention. *Emerg Infect Dis* 1999 Oct.[28] Available from http://www.cdc.gov/ncidod/eid/vol5no5/meltzer.htm

increase in hospitalizations and an 8.2-fold rise in deaths.[30] Clearly, this would outstrip the capacity of the current supply system and place an enormous burden on the supply management for vaccine.[31]

References

1. Sullivan KM. Health impact of influenza in the United States. *Pharmacoeconomics* 1996; **9**(Suppl 3): 26–33.

2. Szucs T. The socio-economic burden of influenza. *J Antimicrob Chemother* 1999; **44**: 11–15.

3. Thompson WW, Shay DK, Weintraub E *et al*. Mortality associated with influenza and respiratory syncytial virus in the United States. *J Am Med Assoc* 2003; **289**: 179–186.

4. US Population Estimates Program at www.census.gov/.

5. Nichol KL, Wuorenma J, von Sternberg T. Benefits of influenza vaccination for low-, intermediate-, and high-risk senior citizens. *Arch Intern Med* 1998; **158**: 1769–1776.

6. Zimmerman R. Lowering the age for routine influenza vaccination to 50 years. *Am Fam Physician* 1999; **60**(7): 2061–2066.

7. Barker WH, Mullooly JP. A study of excess mortality during influenza epidemics in the United States, 1968–1976. *Am J Epidemiol* 1982; **115**: 479–480.

8. Neuzil KM, Wright PF, Mitchel EF, Griffin MR. The burden of influenza illness in children with asthma and other chronic medical conditions. *J Pediatr* 2000; **137**: 856–864.

9. Levy E. French economic evaluations of influenza and influenza vaccination. *Pharmacoeconomics* 1996; **9**(Suppl 3): 62–66.

10. *Statistical Yearbook for Germany*, Frankfurt, 1997.

11. Couch RB. Influenza: prospects for control. *Ann Intern Med* 2000; **133**: 992–998.

12. CDC. Prevention and control of influenza. Recommendations of the Advisory Committee on Immunization Practices (ACIP). *MMWR Recomm Rep* 2001; **50**(RR-4): 1–46.

13. Patriarca PA. New options for prevention and control of influenza. *J Am Med Assoc* 1999; **282**: 75–77.

14. Nichol KL. Cost-benefit analysis of a strategy to vaccinate healthy working adults against influenza. *Arch Intern Med* 2001; **161**(5): 749–759.

15. Elder A, O'Donnell B, McCruden E *et al.* Incidence and recall of influenza in a cohort of Glasgow health care workers during the 1993–4 epidemic: results of serum testing and questionnaire. *Br Med J* 1996; **313**(7067): 1241–1242.

16. Wilde J, MacMillan J, Serwint J *et al.* Effectiveness of influenza vaccine in health care professionals: a randomised trial. *J Am Med Assoc* 1999; **281**: 908–913.

17. Dille JH. A worksite influenza immunization program. Impact on lost work days, health care utilization, and health care spending. *AAOHN J* 1999; **47**(7): 301–309.

18. Mauskopf JA, Cates SC, Griffin AD. A pharmacoeconomic model for the treatment of influenza. *Pharmacoeconomics* 1999; **16**(Suppl 1): 73–84.

19. Bridges C, Thompson W, Melzer M *et al.* Effectiveness and cost-benefit of influenza vaccination of healthy working adults. *J Am Med Assoc* 2000; **284**(13): 1655–1663.

20. Kumpulainen V, Makela M. Influenza vaccination among healthy employees: a cost-benefit analysis. *Scand J Infect Dis* 1997; **29**(2): 181–185.

21. Nichol KL *et al.* The effectiveness of vaccination against influenza in healthy, working adults. *New Engl J Med* 1995; **333**(14): 889–893.

22. Campbell DS, Rumley MH. Cost-effectiveness of the influenza vaccine in a healthy, working-age population. *J Occup Environ Med* 1997; **39**: 408–414

23. Monto AS, Sullivan KM. Acute respiratory illness in the community. Frequency of illness and the agents involved. *Epidemiol Inf* 1993; **110**: 145–160.

24. Keech M, Scott A, Ryan P. The impact of influenza and influenza-like illness on productivity and health care resource

utilisation in a working population. *Occup Med* 1998; **48**(2): 85–90.

25. Burckel E, Ashraf T, Galvao de Sousa Filho J *et al.* Economic impact of providing workplace influenza vaccination. A model and case study application at a Brazilian pharma-chemical company. *Pharmacoeconomics* 1999; **16**(5, Pt 2): 563–576.

26. Neuzil KM *et al.* Illness among schoolchildren during influenza season: effect on school absenteeism, parental absenteeism from work, and secondary illness in families. *Arch Pediatr Adolesc Med* 2002; **156**: 986–991.

27. Barker WH, Borisute H, Cox C. A study of the impact of influenza on the functional status of frail older people. *Arch Intern Med* 1998; **158**: 645–650.

28. Meltzer MI, Cox NJ, Fukuda K. The economic impact of pandemic influenza in the United States: priorities for intervention. Centers for Disease Control and Prevention, Atlanta, Georgia, USA. *Emerg Infect Dis* 1999; **5**(5).

29. Cox NJ, Tamblyn SE, Tam T. Influenza pandemic planning. *Vaccine* 2003; **21**: 1801–1803.

30. Schopflocher DP, Russell ML, Svenson LW, Nguyen TH, Mazurenko I. Pandemic influenza planning: using the U.S. Centers for Disease Control FluAid Software for small area estimation in the Canadian context. *Ann Epidemiol* 2004; **14**: 73–76.

31. Medema JK, Zoellner YF, Ryan J, Palache AM. Modeling pandemic preparedness scenarios: health economic implications of enhanced pandemic vaccine supply. *Virus Res* 2004; **103**: 9–15.

Vaccination: Cornerstone of Influenza Control

Vaccination is the primary and single most cost-effective method of preventing influenza. Flu vaccine development began just a few years after the first isolation of the influenza virus from infected patients in 1933.[1] For an account of the history of influenza vaccine development, see Ref. 2. Initial pioneering studies demonstrated that influenza A/PR/8/34 (H1N1) virus, grown in chicken embryos, would infect humans upon subcutaneous administration, inducing virus-neutralizing antibodies.[2,3] Soon after these first observations, studies using formalin-inactivated H1N1 whole-virus preparations were initiated, the first inactivated influenza vaccines being introduced in the 1940s.[2] Even today, most licensed influenza vaccines are inactivated formulations, consisting of either split virus or subunit preparations containing isolated haemagglutinin (HA) and neuraminidase (NA).[2,4,5] These vaccines are generally produced from virus grown in chicken embryos. Through the application of advanced ultracentrifugation techniques, high degrees of vaccine virus purity are achieved, virtually eliminating any significant adverse effects of the vaccines.

Active immunization against any microbial disease, including influenza, aims at induction of antimicrobial immunity by inoculating the person with an attenuated or inactivated form of the pathogen involved. Following such an approach, one attempts to closely mimic the immune response to a natural infection, which is often considered the "gold standard" for protection. As for influenza, thus far the hallmark for vaccination efficacy has been an adequate level of virus-neutralizing antibodies in the serum.[5–7] These antibodies are primarily directed against the envelope glycoproteins of the virus, HA and NA, HA being the major target for virus-neutralizing antibodies. It is well established that HA-specific antibodies in the circulation protect from severe viral pneumonia as a result of transudation of these antibodies from the blood into the lungs.[6,7]

Current influenza vaccines contain antigens from two influenza A virus strains and one B strain, according to annual recommendation by the WHO.[8,9] To ensure an optimal antigenic match between the virus strains in the vaccine and the viruses circulating in the subsequent influenza season, this WHO recommendation is based on intensive surveillance of new influenza strains around the globe, allowing an informed selection of strains to be included in the next annual vaccine.[8,9] Today, many countries have implemented influenza vaccination programmes, the primary target groups for vaccination including the elderly and people with underlying medical conditions which make them vulnerable to serious complications of influenza.[9–11] Also, there is increasing awareness of the potential societal and health benefits of vaccinating working adults and children.

Current inactivated influenza vaccines have an excellent safety record.[9,12] Hundreds of millions of vaccine doses are distributed worldwide each year, adverse effects being extremely rare. Influenza vaccination has been shown to be highly effective. Vaccination results in reductions of influenza-related respiratory illness and number of physician visits among all age groups, and in lower hospitalization rates and deaths among the elderly and patients at risk for serious complications of influenza.[13,14] Vaccination coverage among target groups has increased considerably in recent years[10] as the awareness of the impact of influenza is growing, and influenza has become an important issue on the public health agenda in many countries.[15,16] However, the use of available influenza vaccines is still far from optimal. Primary-care physicians are in a key position to explain the favourable benefit–risk ratio of influenza vaccination to people in target groups and motivate them to take the vaccine. Increased use of influenza vaccines is expected to significantly reduce epidemics and to improve our preparedness for potential new pandemic outbreaks.

Key Messages
• Current inactivated influenza vaccines have an excellent safety record.
• Influenza vaccination results in significant reductions in influenza-related respiratory illness, hospitalization rates and deaths among the elderly and patients at risk for serious complications of influenza.
• Influenza vaccination of the elderly and patients with underlying medical conditions is cost-effective and in many cases cost-saving.
• Scientific evidence also demonstrates the benefits of vaccinating healthy working adults and children.
• Misconceptions about the benefits of influenza vaccination and overestimation of its risks lead to decreased acceptance and suboptimal use of influenza vaccines.
• Primary-care physicians play a pivotal role in explaining the favourable benefit–risk ratio of influenza vaccination and in motivating patients in target groups to take the vaccinaton.
• The WHO strongly supports increased use of influenza vaccine among the elderly and people in other target groups.

Current inactivated influenza vaccines

Vaccine formulations

Initial inactivated influenza vaccine formulations invariably consisted of whole inactivated virus formulations, the virus being produced in chicken embryos.[2,4] Whole inactivated virus vaccines are generally quite immunogenic. However, despite the improved techniques for virus purification, local reactogenicity and systemic side-effects remain a problem associated with the use of these vaccines, particularly in small children.[17] This has led to the introduction of vaccine formulations consisting of disrupted virus particles, which turned out to be almost equally immunogenic, in terms of induction of antibody responses in primed individuals, yet causing significantly fewer side-effects. These split-virus vaccines, first licensed in the USA in 1968, are among the most widely used formulations to date. While ether was the original splitting agent of choice, currently detergents such as Tween 80, Triton N101, cetyl trimethyl ammonium bromide (CTAB) and sodium deoxycholate are used in addition to ether to disrupt the virus particles.[4] A disadvantage of split vaccines, relative to whole inactivated virus, is their comparatively low immunogenicity in unprimed individuals, such as young children without prior exposure to flu virus or vaccine, requiring a booster immunization for adequate protection.[18]

Relative to split-virus vaccines, subunit preparations represent a further refinement and improvement of the vaccine formulation. Subunit vaccines contain the HA and NA surface glycoproteins of the virus purified from other viral components.[4] Because of their high purity, subunit vaccines have a favourable profile in terms of local and systemic side-effects, compared to whole-virus and split vaccines.[19] However, subunit vaccines are equally immunogenic in primed individuals. The concept of using just the isolated viral HA and NA antigens is based on the notion that the primary correlate of protection against influenza is an adequate level of circulating antibodies against the surface glycoproteins of the virus, especially HA. Surface glycoproteins used in subunit vaccines are isolated after splitting of the virus by detergent treatment, and subsequent removal of the detergent through adsorption on a hydrophobic resin such as Amberlite. This process results in the formation of rosettes of HA and NA, with only small amounts of contaminating core proteins, such as NP or M1, or viral membrane lipid.[4] Influenza subunit vaccines were first licensed in UK in 1980 and are now used in many countries worldwide.

Selection of vaccine strains

To be effective, the vaccine components need to match those of the circulating influenza virus strains in the target season. Current influenza vaccines contain three virus strains, two A strains (an H3N2 and an H1N1 strain) and one B strain. These strains are included in the vaccines on recommendation of the WHO.[8,9] This recommendation is based on an extensive review of epidemiological data and antigenic and genetic analyses of virus isolates by the four WHO Collaborating Centres. In order to allow vaccine manufacturers sufficient time for production, in February of each year the WHO issues its recommendation about which viral strains should be included in the next winter's vaccine for the northern hemisphere. A second review follows in September to consider adjustments of the vaccine composition for the southern hemisphere.

That this system of surveillance and recommendation, in fact, works quite well is demonstrated by the good match achieved in, for example, the influenza seasons from 1987 to 1997.[5] Within this period, 23 vaccine strains recommended by the WHO matched with the subsequently circulating total of 30 virus strains (Table 14). A complete match of all three strains was achieved in five out of 10 seasons. Nevertheless, an intrinsic uncertainty remains and sometimes there is not a perfect match between vaccine strain and circulating virus, in which case the vaccine may have reduced efficacy. However, these occasional mismatches should by no means be regarded as a justification for not providing or taking the vaccination.

Dose standardization

The development of the single radial immunodiffusion (SRD) test has allowed the implementation of a stringent standardization of vaccine dosaging.[5] The SRD test determines the content of HA antigen in influenza vaccines on the basis of the immunological activity of the antigen against a reference sheep antiserum (Figure 23).[5] The application of this assay and the use of standardized

Match between vaccine recommendations and concurrent epidemic influenza virus strains			
Season	**A/H1N1**	**A/H3N2**	**B**
1987–1988	+	–	–
1988–1989	+	+	+
1989–1990	+	+	+
1990–1991	+	–	+
1991–1992	+	+	+
1992–1993	+	–	+
1993–1994	+	–	+
1994–1995	+	–	–
1995–1996	+	+	+
1996–1997	+	+	+

Table 14. Match between WHO vaccine recommendations and epidemic virus strains circulating in subsequent winter season. Adapted from Wood JM. Standardization of inactivated influenza vaccines. In: Nicholson KG, Webster RG, Hay AJ, editors. *Textbook of Influenza*. Blackwell Science, 1998; pp. 333–345[5] with permission from Blackwell Publishing.

reagents, supplied by one of the WHO Collaborating Centres to influenza vaccine manufacturers, thus guarantee optimal uniformity among different influenza vaccine formulations in terms of potency.[5]

Several studies have shown that a vaccine dose of >10 μg HA per strain would generally induce an adequate immune response in primed individuals.[20,21] Current trivalent inactivated influenza vaccines contain 15 μg of HA per strain as assessed by the SRD assay. This dose scheme has been formally standardized.[5,22,23] The trivalent inactivated influenza vaccine is administered by intramuscular or deep subcutaneous injection.

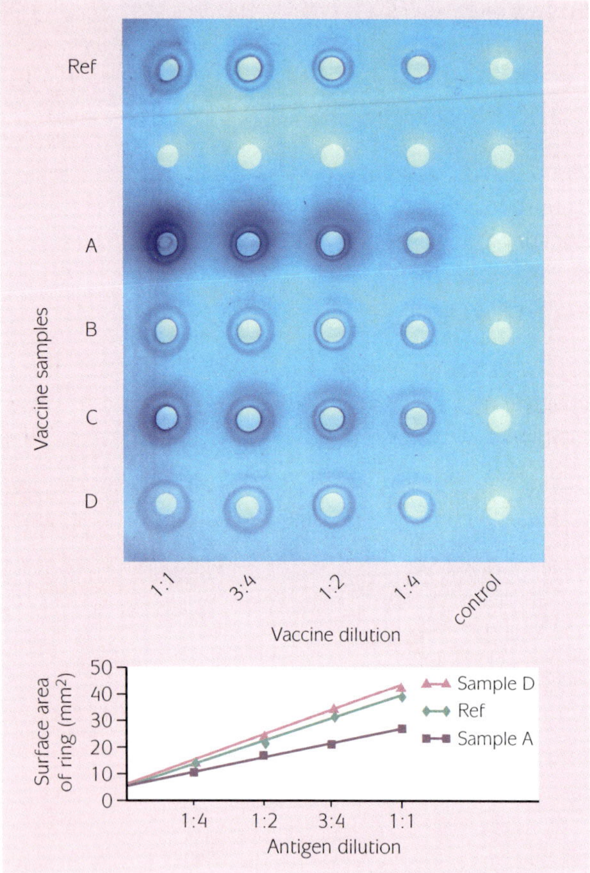

Figure 23. Single radial immunodiffusion (SRD) test of influenza vaccine potency.[5] Serial dilutions of detergent-treated vaccine, and a reference antigen (Ref), are added to wells in an agarose gel containing a sheep antiserum against the relevant HA. The surface area of the precipitation rings formed (top) is subsequently plotted as a function of the dilution of the vaccine (bottom). The slope of the resulting curves is a direct measure of the HA concentration in the vaccine, and is compared with that of the reference curve. In the graph, data for vaccine samples A and D and the reference antigen shown in the top gel are plotted. Courtesy of Jeroen Medema, Solvay Pharmaceuticals, Weesp, the Netherlands.

Evaluation of vaccine immunogenicity

Not only has the composition of influenza vaccines been standardized in many countries, in the EU criteria for vaccine immunogenicity have also been implemented.[5,22,23] As indicated above, current inactivated influenza vaccines aim at induction of an efficient systemic antibody response against the viral surface antigens, primarily HA. Accordingly, vaccine efficacy is evaluated on the basis of serological data, in particular seroprotection rates and antibody titres.

Antibody titres are generally determined on the basis of haemagglutination–inhibition (HI) activity[5,6] or, occasionally, by single radial haemolysis (SRH).[5] In the HI assay, serum samples of vaccinated individuals are tested for their ability

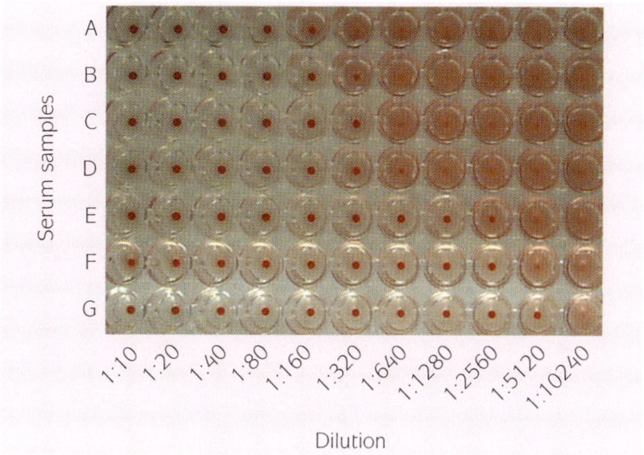

Figure 24. Haemagglutination–inhibition (HI) titration of an antiserum against influenza. Turkey or guinea pig erythrocytes are incubated with a standard amount of influenza virus and two-fold dilutions of the serum to be evaluated. The reciprocal of the highest dilution at which haemagglutination is completely inhibited (haemagglutination inhibition is observed as the formation of a small concentrated dot of red cells in the bottom of the well) is defined as the HI titre of the sample. For example, the HI titre of serum C is 320, that of serum F is 2560. Courtesy of René Benne, Regional Public Health Laboratory, Groningen, the Netherlands.

European Union criteria for the assessment of vaccines		
Criterion	**18–60 years**	**>60 years**
Seroconversions or significant rises in anti-HA antibody titre	>40%	>30%
Mean geometric increase in titre	>2.5	>2.0
Patients achieving HI titre ≥ 40 or SRH titre >25 mm²	>70%	>60%

For each virus strain, at least one of the above criteria should be met

Table 15. Criteria of the European Medicines Agency (EMEA) of the EU for the evaluation of influenza vaccine efficacy. Issued by the Committee on Proprietary Medicinal Products (CPMP). Note for guidance on harmonization of requirements for influenza vaccines. CPMP/BWP/214/96, 1997 (http://www.emea.eu.int/pdfs/human/bwp/021496en.pdf)[22] ©EMEA 1997 Reproduction and/or distribution of this document is authorised for non-commercial purposes only provided the EMEA is acknowledged.

to inhibit agglutination of erythrocytes, induced by influenza virus through interaction of the viral HA with sialic acid-containing glycoproteins and glycolipids on the red cell surface. Antibodies directed against HA interfere with this interaction, thus inhibiting the agglutination process. In practice, serial dilutions of serum are incubated with a standardized amount of influenza virus, after which a fixed concentration of erythrocytes, generally from guinea-pigs or turkeys, is added and the extent of haemagglutination determined. The highest serum dilution at which agglutination still occurs is defined as the HI titre (Figure 24). The SRH test evaluates the capacity of serial dilutions of antibodies against HA to lyse erythrocytes in the presence of guinea-pig complement.[5]

The European Medicines Agency (EMEA) has formally standardized the EU requirements for annual evaluation of influenza vaccine efficacy (Table 15).[22,23] These requirement include specificied levels of titre increase or numbers of significant increases in antibody titre upon vaccination. In addition, there is the requirement for an annual clinical study among 50 volunteers of 18–60 years of age and above 60 years.

Annual timetable for vaccine production and licensing

As almost all current influenza vaccines are prepared from egg-grown virus (Figure 25), the annual vaccine production cycle begins with the estimation and ordering of the required numbers of chicken embryos well before actual vaccine production starts.[24] Then, after the WHO has issued its recommendation, high-growth reassortant seed viruses are generated and characterized for approval by the WHO Collaborating Centres. These seed viruses are high-growth reassortants (see pp. 45–67), carrying the HA and NA of the recommended vaccine virus on a background of a virus that replicates well in chicken embryos. Generally, 1–2 months after the WHO recommendation, seed virus lots are released to the manufacturers. Vaccine production then

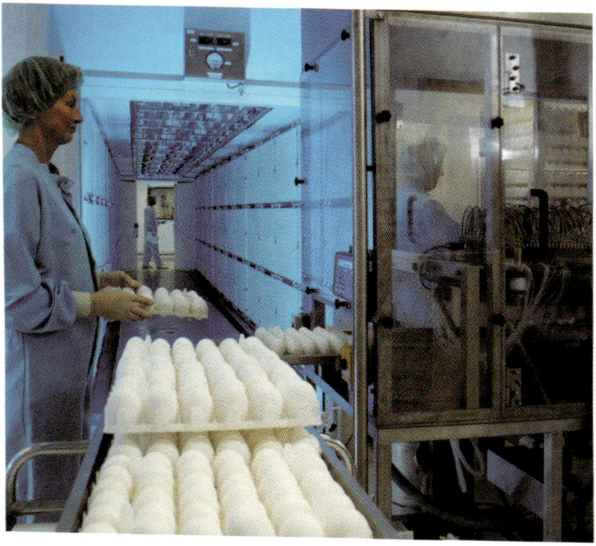

Figure 25. Production of influenza vaccine virus on chicken embryos. Courtesy of Solvay Pharmaceuticals, Weesp, the Netherlands.

continues for several months. In this process, quantification of the potency of monovalent vaccine bulks is a critical step, requiring the availability of specific reagents for SRD determination. Finally, the ultimate trivalent vaccine can be formulated and the syringes filled. Immediately after the first batches of trivalent vaccine have been produced, tested and released for use, two serological clinical studies (in people aged 18–60 and >60 years) are performed to satisfy the licensing criteria of the European regulatory authorities,[22,23] as discussed above. Results of these clinical studies form part of the annual registration dossier for market authorization in the member states of the EU.

From the time of recommendation by the WHO of virus strains to be included in the vaccine, there is an approximate 6-month period to bring the vaccine to the market. Within two campaigns for the northern and southern hemispheres, a total of about 290 million doses of influenza vaccine are currently being produced each year (D. Fedson, Influenza Vaccine Supply Task Force, unpublished data).

Recommendations and vaccination coverage

For a long time, doubts and misconceptions about the benefit–risk ratio of influenza vaccination have hampered the implementation of recommended policies for influenza vaccination. However, in recent years, influenza vaccination has become a prominent issue on the public health agenda of an increasing number of countries. Many developed as well as developing countries have now adopted formal recommendations on influenza vaccination for specific target groups. Although still a matter of national responsibility, these recommendations have become increasingly uniform, particularly throughout Western Europe, and in North America, Australia, New Zealand and Japan. In addition, in 2000, the WHO has issued for the first time a formal recommendation for the use of inactivated vaccines for the prevention of influenza.[9]

Recommendations for influenza vaccination

Table 16 presents the recommendations for influenza vaccination adopted in most countries. The elderly represent the primary target group.[10,11] This recommendation follows the increased susceptibility of the elderly for infectious diseases in general, which may be explained, at least partly, by a gradual decline in immune competence with age, particularly at the level of T-cell function (see pp. 68–85). The recommendation is also based

Influenza vaccination recommendations in European countries
• People aged >65 years.
• Residents of nursing homes and other long-term care facilities.
• Adults and children with chronic pulmonary disorders.
• Adults and children with chronic cardiovascular disorders.
• Those who have required regular medical follow-up or hospitalization during the preceding year because of – chronic metabolic diseases (including diabetes mellitus), – renal dysfunction, – haemoglobinopathies, or – immunosuppression (including immunosuppression caused by medications or by human immunodeficiency virus).
• Children and teenagers (aged 6 months to 18 years) who are receiving long-term aspirin therapy and therefore might be at risk for developing Reye's syndrome after influenza infection.
• Vaccination of health care workers and others in close contact with persons at high risk, including household members, is recommended.

Table 16. Recommendations for influenza vaccination adopted in most European countries. Adapted from Van Essen GA *et al.* Influenza vaccination in 2000: vaccination recommendations and vaccine use in 50 developed and developing countries. *Vaccine* 2003; **21**: 1780–1785[10] with permission from Elsevier.

on the proven clinical effectiveness of flu vaccination of the elderly. In most countries, flu vaccination is recommended for all individuals above 60 or 65 years of age. In a few countries, including the USA and Belgium, the limit has been set at 50 years due to the increased prevalence of high-risk conditions for influenza illness among people over 50. Vaccination is also quite uniformly recommended for individuals with specific medical conditions, including cardiovascular, pulmonary and renal disease, diabetes and immunodeficiency.[10] In addition, many countries recommend flu vaccination for nursing-home residents, health care workers and household contacts of high-risk individuals.[10]

Current use of influenza vaccines

Along with the implementation of formal recommendations for flu vaccination in an increasing number of countries, the use of influenza vaccine has increased considerably in the last decade or so.[10] The most dramatic changes in this respect have occurred in Latin America and the central and eastern countries in Europe. Figure 26 presents a survey of influenza vaccine use in 40 developed and rapidly developing countries in the year 2002.

As mentioned above, the total number of influenza vaccine doses distributed annually worldwide, has increased in recent years to an estimated level of 290 million in 2004. About 30% of these doses goes to North America, and an approximately equal fraction to Western Europe.[10] Importantly, in the year 2000, about one-third of the total number of vaccine doses was used in countries outside Western Europe, North America, Australia and New Zealand.[10] This trend indicates that developing countries are

Figure 26. Use of influenza vaccine in 40 developed and developing countries in the year 2002. Data from Macroepidemiology of Influenza Vaccination Study Group. Adapted and updated from van Essen GA *et al*. Influenza vaccination in 2000: recommendations and vaccine use in 50 developed and rapidly developing countries. *Vaccine* 2003; **21**(16): 1780–1785 with permission from Elsevier.

also beginning to implement measures for influenza prevention and control on an annual basis.

However, despite the increased vaccination coverage among target groups, the use of influenza vaccine is still

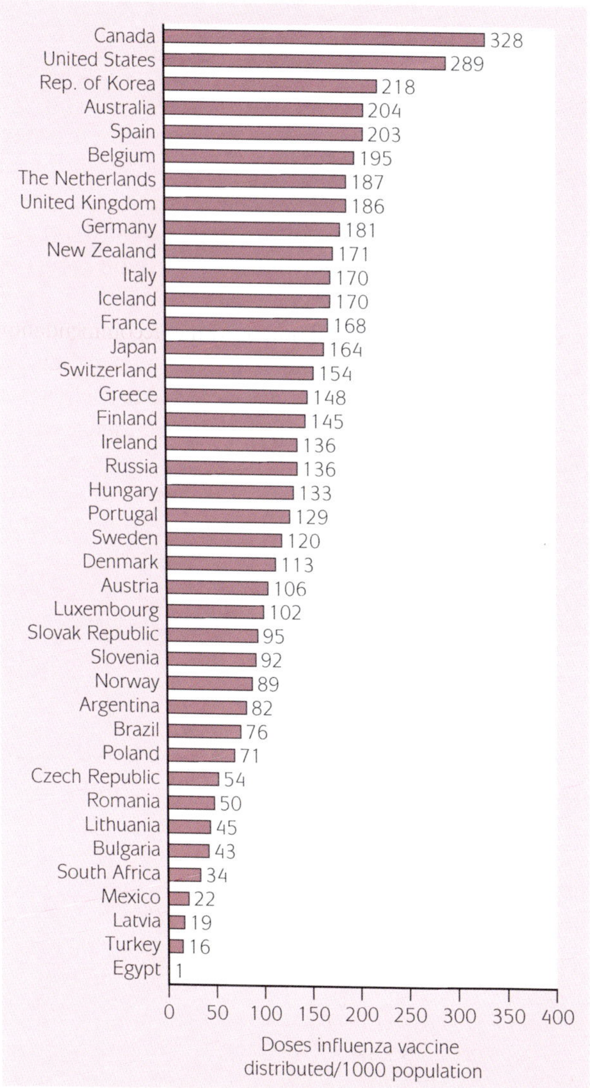

far from optimal in many countries. The single most important factor influencing the use of influenza vaccine is whether it is recommended by the doctor. Therefore, primary-care physicians play an important major role in implementing influenza vaccination programmes, as discussed in more detail on pages 166–189.

Benefits of influenza vaccination

The value of immunization against influenza has long been questioned, as outbreaks of flu continue despite increased influenza vaccination coverage. Therefore, there has been a demand for sound scientific data on the effects of influenza vaccination. Many clinical studies have produced consistent results showing clear-cut benefits of influenza vaccination.[13,14] Since the elderly comprise by far the largest target population for flu vaccination, the majority of studies evaluating the benefits of vaccination have been conducted among people in this age group; these will be discussed in more detail below. Individual studies have also indicated clear-cut beneficial effects in other target groups, such as diabetics and patients with asthma or cardiovascular disease. In addition, there is increasing evidence and awareness of the potential benefits of influenza vaccination of younger healthy (working) adults[13,14] and children.[13]

Vaccine efficacy and clinical effectiveness of influenza vaccination

In evaluating the outcome of influenza vaccination, a distinction is often made between vaccine efficacy *per se* and the clinical effectiveness of vaccination.[13,14] Vaccine efficacy is defined as the reduction in the rate of laboratory-confirmed influenza among vaccinated compared to non-vaccinated individuals. Vaccine efficacy thus provides a direct measure of the specific reduction in influenza infection rates as a result of the vaccination. With an approximate annual attack rate of influenza of 5–10%, accurate determination of vaccine efficacy requires well-controlled studies and evaluation of large study groups.

Obviously, vaccine efficacy will depend critically on the match between the vaccine components and the circulating virus strains.

Clinical effectiveness provides a less specific, yet quite relevant and important, measure of the benefit of influenza vaccination. It is defined as the reduction of clinically relevant, but not necessarily influenza-specific, disease in a "real-life" situation, including all influenza-like illness, hospitalizations due to pneumonia from all causes or death from all causes.[13,14] As this parameter includes – by definition – disease outcomes that are not caused by the influenza virus, clinical effectiveness of vaccination is generally estimated to be lower than the actual vaccine efficacy, as illustrated by the hypothetical example presented in Figure 27.[14] Therefore, clinical effectiveness should not be confused for vaccine efficacy, as this may result in a substantial underestimation of the actual performance of the vaccine.

Health benefits of vaccination of the elderly

Several studies have indicated that, in cases of a good match between vaccine strain and circulating virus, the efficacy of current inactivated influenza vaccines among the elderly is approximately 60%. For example, in a large, randomized, double-blind, placebo-controlled trial among 1838 subjects of 60 years of age or older in the Netherlands, vaccine efficacy was found to be 58%.[25] This trial was conducted in the 1991–92 winter season and involved the use of a multivalent inactivated influenza vaccine, matching well with the circulating virus.

Numerous studies have convincingly demonstrated the clinical benefits of influenza vaccination in the elderly.[13,14] For example, in a large study in the USA, spanning two influenza seasons (1998–2000) and involving 300,000 community-dwelling elderly people (≥65 years old), influenza vaccination was performed in 55.5–59.7% of the population. The vaccination was associated with significant reductions in pneumonia (29–32%), cardiac disease (19%)

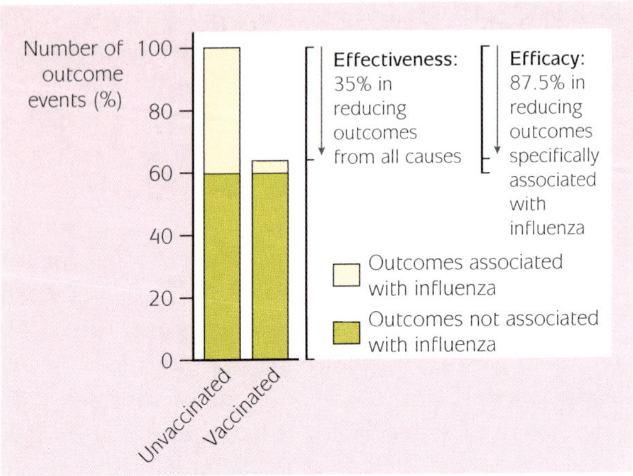

Figure 27. Relationship between influenza vaccine efficacy and clinical effectiveness of influenza vaccination. The figure shows a hypothetical example in which vaccination is associated with a 35% reduction in all outcomes evaluated (such as hospitalizations for pneumonia). However, not all outcomes are due to influenza. If only 40% of the outcomes represented complications of influenza, the underlying efficacy of the vaccine preventing direct influenza-associated outcomes would be 35%/0.4 = 87.5%. Adapted from Nichol KL. Efficacy/clinical effectiveness of inactivated influenza virus vaccines in adults. In: Nicholson KG, Webster RG, Hay AJ, editors. *Textbook of Influenza*. Blackwell Science, 1998; pp. 358–372[14] with permission from Blackwell Publishing.

and cerebrovascular disease (16–23%).[26] Other studies have indicated that influenza vaccination of patients who have had a myocardial infarction results in a significant reduction in 1-year mortality rates (66% reduction) or risk of further ischaemic events. A meta-analysis, including a large number of individual studies among senior citizens living in the community, concluded that vaccination significantly reduces hospitalization and death rates among the elderly (Table 17).[27] Another meta-analysis has shown that influenza vaccination is also highly effective among residents of nursing homes (Table 17).[28] These findings highlight the

Clinical effectiveness of influenza vaccination of the elderly	
Outcome measure	**Reduction**
Community-dwelling senior citizens	
Hospitalizations for	
Pneumonia from all causes	33%
All respiratory conditions	32%
Congestive heart failure	27%
Death from all causes	50%
Elderly in nursing homes	
Respiratory illness	56%
Pneumonia from all causes	53%
Hospitalization in general	48%
Death from all causes	68%

Table 17. Clinical effectiveness of influenza vaccination of the elderly. Adapted from Nichol KL. The efficacy, effectiveness and cost-effectiveness of inactivated influenza virus vaccines. *Vaccine* 2003; **21**: 1769–1775[13] with permission from Elsevier.

benefits of influenza vaccination of the elderly and support efforts to increase the rate of vaccination in this target group.

Cost-effectiveness of vaccination of the elderly

Economic evaluations, conducted in many different countries, have indicated that vaccination of senior citizens against influenza is always cost-effective and frequently cost-saving.[13,14] For example, in a 6-year study carried out in Minnesota, influenza vaccination of nursing home residents was associated with an average net saving of US $73 per person as a result of reductions in direct medical costs.[29] Vaccination appears to be cost-effective or even cost-saving for both healthy senior citizens and high-risk elderly with underlying chronic medical conditions. In a study conducted in the Netherlands in the 1995–96 and

1997–98 seasons, influenza vaccination was found to be cost-saving for high-risk elderly and cost-effective for all elderly and elderly at low risk, the cost-effectiveness ratios being €1820 per life-year gained for all elderly and €6900 per life-year gained for those at low risk.[30] Similar studies have been conducted in, for example, France and Germany with comparable outcomes.

Vaccination of healthy younger adults

While younger adults are generally not at risk for serious complications due to influenza, flu remains an important cause of work absenteeism, diminished work productivity and malaise interfering with off-work activities. This is why there is an increasing awareness of the potential benefits of vaccination of working adults.[13,14] Several prospective clinical studies have demonstrated the efficacy of inactivated influenza vaccines among healthy younger adults. Initial trials, conducted among military recruits several decades ago, showed that the vaccine was 70–90% efficacious in preventing laboratory-confirmed influenza, provided there was a good antigenic match between vaccine and circulating virus. A review of more recent clinical studies shows that the efficacy of inactivated influenza vaccines varies from 65% for all influenza seasons to 72% for those seasons where there was a good match between vaccine and circulating virus.[31] Additional studies have reported vaccine efficacies in terms of prevention of confirmed influenza in the range of 80–90% in cases where there was a good match.[32,33] Clearly, current inactivated influenza vaccines attain very high efficacy values among healthy younger adults (Table 18).

As demonstrated by a number of studies, conducted in different countries, vaccination significantly reduces illness, absenteeism and influenza-related costs for healthy adults in the workplace.[13,14] For example, vaccination reduces upper respiratory tract and influenza-like illnesses from all causes by approximately 30%, related physician visits by >40% and work loss by >35% (Table 18).[33,34]

Would there then be an economic benefit associated with routine vaccination of healthy working adults? Cost-benefit analyses, based on clinical trials or on modelling, have shown that vaccination of healthy working adults is cost-effective and in many cases cost-saving, provided that indirect costs associated with work absenteeism are explicitly taken into account. For example, trials conducted in the USA have shown that – with an average cost for vaccine production and administration of $20 – the net saving would be $23 per person vaccinated.[35] In another study comparing 131 vaccinated employees from six textile plants in North Carolina, USA, with 131 age- and gender-matched non-vaccinated controls from different plants, the "cost per saved lost workday" was $22.36, resulting in an overall saving of $2.58 per dollar invested in the vaccination programme.[36] Other, model-based, studies also indicate that vaccinating working adults would be cost-saving.[13] Even

Benefits of influenza vaccination of healthy adults and children	
Outcome measure	**Reduction (%)**
Healthy adults <65 years of age	
Laboratory-confirmed influenza	70–90
URI/ILI (all causes)	25–34
Work loss due to URI/ILI	32–43
Physician visits due to URI/ILI	42–44
Children	
Laboratory-confirmed influenza	60–90
Acute otitis media (all causes)	30–36

Table 18. Benefits of influenza vaccination of healthy adults and children. ILI, influenza-like illness; URI, upper respiratory illness. Adapted from Nichol KL. The efficacy, effectiveness and cost-effectiveness of inactivated influenza virus vaccines. *Vaccine* 2003; **21**: 1769–1775[13] with permission from Elsevier.

when indirect costs are not taken into account, vaccination of adults below the age of 65 turns out to be highly cost-effective. For example, a cost-utility analysis of the US Office of Technology Assessment found that a year of healthy life gained would cost $278 per person of 25–44 years of age and only $100 for those 45–64 years old.[37]

Vaccination of children

Even though, in most countries, children are not included in the target groups, they are increasingly under consideration for routine flu vaccination.[13] It is generally accepted that children play an important role in the spread of influenza infections in communities. In addition, influenza among children is a significant cause of parental work loss. Furthermore, very small children may well be at increased risk for serious influenza-associated complications. For this reason, the Advisory Committee on Immunization Practices (ACIP) in the USA has encouraged routine vaccination of children of 6–23 months of age.[38]

The efficacy of influenza vaccination among children has been evaluated in a number of randomized, controlled trials, involving the use of either trivalent inactivated or experimental live-attenuated vaccines.[39,40] From these studies, it appears that vaccination is highly efficacious in terms of preventing laboratory-confirmed influenza for children in their teens (~90%), whereas a lower efficacy is seen with younger children (Table 18). For example, an Italian study among children 1–6 years of age showed a reduction by 67% in influenza-like illness. Other studies generally confirm this picture.[40] The comparatively modest immunogenicity of influenza vaccines among small children is probably due to their lack of pre-exposure to either influenza virus or vaccine. Therefore, for these immunologically naive children, usually a two-dose vaccination regimen is recommended.

A common complication of influenza among young children is acute otitis media. There appears to be a clear-cut benefit associated with influenza vaccination in terms of reducing the incidence of otitis media. A clinical study conducted in Finland, for example, has demonstrated a reduction of 36% in overall rate of otitis media as a result of vaccination (Table 18), which corresponded to an 83% reduction among children with laboratory-confirmed influenza.[41]

Another benefit of vaccinating children relates to the associated prevention of secondary transmission among family members or others within the neighbourhood. In a study conducted in Michigan, USA, during the 1968–69 pandemic outbreak of Hong Kong flu, vaccination of school-age children resulted in three-fold lower rates of influenza-like illness than in a control community.[42] Interestingly, a 20-year programme in Japan, involving vaccination of school-age children, has indicated that there may be a correlation between increased vaccination of children and lower excess mortality among the elderly,[43] substantiating the notion that vaccination of children reduces secondary influenza transmission.

Finally, vaccination of children appears to be highly cost-effective and in many cases cost-saving. The analysis by the US Office of Technology Assessment, referred to above,[37] indicates that vaccination of children below 3 years of age would cost US $1122 per year of healthy life gained, while vaccinating children 3–14 years of age would only cost US $853 per year of healthy life gained. More recent analyses of influenza vaccination of children also clearly indicate its economic benefits.[44] Even at an average cost of influenza vaccine production and administration of US $20, vaccination of children is likely to be cost-saving, part of the benefit in this respect being due to a reduction in parental work loss.[13] Accordingly, some health authorities start to expand the recommended use of influenza vaccines to include young children as well as other groups, as discussed in more detail in the final chapter of this book.

Vaccine safety and contraindications

Current inactivated influenza vaccines, the split-virus and subunit formulations in particular, have an excellent safety record.[9,12] Hundreds of millions of vaccine doses are being administered annually around the globe, and the overall rate of adverse reactions is extremely low. However, sporadically, adverse reactions do occur. These include, in particular, local reactions at the site of injection.[12] Generally, the reactions are mild and of a transient nature. It has also been clearly demonstrated that influenza vaccination of patients with asthma is safe. In a large, double-blind, placeco-controlled study, it was demonstrated that no exacerbation of asthma occurred as a result of vaccination.[45]

It is important to note that there is no vaccination procedure, or even medical intervention in general, that bears no risks whatsoever. The same is true for influenza vaccination. However, clearly, the benefits of influenza vaccination by far outweigh its risks. Nevertheless, there are widespread misconceptions regarding the benefit–risk ratio of influenza vaccination. Indeed, some vaccinated individuals even complain of having acquired "the flu" as a result of the vaccination. Primary-care physicians have the responsibility to give their patients a proper view of the favourable benefit–risk ratio of influenza vaccination.

In specific subpopulations, influenza vaccination is contraindicated. These include people with hypersensitivity to eggs and/or a history of immediate allergic reactions following the vaccination. Allergic reactions to flu vaccination are most likely due to the presence of traces of egg-derived components in the vaccine, ovalbumin in particular. Novel developments, specifically the production of vaccine virus by cell culture technology, should eliminate this problem. Vaccination is also contraindicated in patients with a history of Guillain–Barré syndrome (GBS). There have been reports about a possible association between GBS and influenza vaccination, particularly during the swine flu vaccination campaign in the USA in 1976–77.[46] More recent studies suggest that GBS may occur at a very low rate of about one additional case per million vaccinees.[47]

References

1. Smith W, Andrews CH, Laidlaw PP. A virus obtained from influenza patients. *Lancet* 1933; **ii**: 66–68.

2. Wood JM, Williams MS. History of inactivated influenza vaccines. In: Nicholson KG, Webster RG, Hay AJ, editors. *Textbook of Influenza*. Blackwell Science, 1998; pp. 317–323.

3. Francis T, Magill TP. The incidence of neutralizing antibodies for human influenza virus in the serum of human individuals of different ages. *J Exp Med* 1936; **63**: 655–668.

4. Furminger IGS. Vaccine production. In: Nicholson KG, Webster RG, Hay AJ, editors. *Textbook of Influenza*. Blackwell Science, 1998; pp. 324–332.

5. Wood JM. Standardization of inactivated influenza vaccines. In: Nicholson KG, Webster RG, Hay AJ, editors. *Textbook of Influenza*. Blackwell Science, 1998; pp. 333–345.

6. Hobson D, Curry RL, Beare AS, Ward-Gardner A. The role of serum haemagglutination-inhibiting antibody in protection against challenge virus infection with A2 and B viruses. *J Hyg (Lond)* 1972; **70**: 767–777.

7. Small PR, Waldman RA, Bruono JC, Gifford GE. Influenza infection in ferrets: Role of serum antibody in protection and recovery. *Infect Immun* 1976; **13**: 417–424.

8. Ghendon,Y. Influenza surveillance. *Bull World Health Org* 1991; **61**: 509–515.

9. World Health Organization. Influenza vaccines. *Wkly Epidemiol Rec* 2000; **75**: 281–288.

10. Van Essen GA, Forleo E, Palache AM, Fedson DS. Influenza vaccination in 2000: vaccination recommendations and vaccine use in 50 developed and developing countries. *Vaccine* 2003; **21**: 1780–1785.

11. World Health Organization. Influenza vaccines. *Wkly Epidemiol Rec* 2002; **77**: 230–239.

12. Wiselka MJ. Vaccine safety. In: Nicholson KG, Webster RG, Hay AJ, editors. *Textbook of Influenza*. Blackwell Science, 1998; pp. 346–357.

13. Nichol KL. The efficacy, effectiveness and cost-effectiveness of inactivated influenza virus vaccines. *Vaccine* 2003; **21**: 1769–1775.

14. Nichol KL. Efficacy/clinical effectiveness of inactivated influenza virus vaccines in adults. In: Nicholson KG, Webster RG, Hay AJ, editors. *Textbook of Influenza*. Blackwell Science, 1998; pp. 358–372.

15. Stöhr K. The global agenda on influenza surveillance and control. *Vaccine* 2003; **21**: 1744–1748.

16. World Health Organization. Global agenda on influenza – adopted version. Part I, *Wkly Epidemiol Rec* 2002; **77**: 179–182; Part II, *Wkly Epidemiol Rec* 2002; **77**: 191–196 (http://www.who.int/emc/diseases/flu/global_agenda_report/Contentpandemic.htm)

17. Ruben FL. Prevention and control of influenza. Role of vaccine. *Am J Med* 1987; **82**(Suppl 6a): 31–34.

18. Nicholson KG, Tyrrell DAJ, Harrison P *et al*. Clinical studies of monovalent inactivated whole virus and subunit A/USSR/77 (H1N1) vaccine: serological responses and clinical reactions. *J Biol Stand* 1979; **7**: 123–136.

19. Beyer WEP, Palache AM, Osterhaus ADME. Comparison of serology and reactogenicity between influenza subunit vaccines and whole or split vaccines. A review and meta-analysis of the literature. *Clin Drug Invest* 1998; **15**: 1–12.

20. Palache AM, Beyer WEP, Lüchters G *et al*. Influenza vaccines: the effect of vaccine dose on antibody response in primed populations during the ongoing interpandemic period. A review of the literature. *Vaccine* 1993; **11**: 892–908.

21. Treanor J, Keitel W, Belshe R, *et al*. Evaluation of a single dose of half strength inactivated influenza vaccine in healthy adults. *Vaccine* 2002; **20**: 1099–1105.

22. European Medicines Agency (EMEA). Note for guidance on harmonization of requirements for influenza vaccines. CPMP/BWP/214/96, 1997 (http://www.emea.eu.int/pdfs/human/bwp/021496en.pdf)

23. Wood JM, Levandowski RA. The influenza vaccine

licensing process. *Vaccine* 2003; **21**: 1786–1788.

24. Gerdil C. The annual production cycle for influenza vaccine. *Vaccine* 2003; **21**: 1776–1779.

25. Govaert TME, Thijs CTMCN, Masurel N *et al.* The efficacy of influenza vaccination in elderly individuals. A randomized double-blind placebo-controlled trial. *J Am Med Assoc* 1994; **272**: 1661–1665.

26. Nichol KL, Nordin J, Mullooly J *et al.* Influenza vaccination and reduction in hospitalizations for cardiac disease and stroke among the elderly. *New Engl J Med* 2003; **348**: 1322–1332.

27. Vu T, Farish S, Jenkins M, Kelly H. A meta-analysis of effectiveness of influenza vaccine in persons aged 65 years and over living in the community. *Vaccine* 2002; **20**: 1831–1836.

28. Gross PA, Hermogenes AW, Sachs HS, Lau J, Levandowski RA. The efficacy of influenza vaccine in elderly persons: a meta-analysis and review of the literature. *Ann Intern Med* 1995; **123**: 518–527.

29. Nichol KL, Wuornema J, Von Sternberg T. Benefits of influenza vaccination for low-, intermediate- and high-risk senior citizens. *Arch Intern Med* 1998; **158**: 1769–1776.

30. Postma MJ, Bos JM, Van Gennip M *et al.* Economic evaluation of influenza vaccination. Assessment for The Netherlands. *Pharmacoeconomics* 1999; **16**(Suppl 1): 33–40.

31. Demicheli V, Jefferson T, Rivetti D, Deeks J. Prevention and early treatment of influenza in healthy adults. *Vaccine* 2000; **18**: 957–1030.

32. Wilde JA, McMillan JA, Serwint J *et al.* Effectiveness of influenza vaccine in health care professionals: a randomized trial. *J Am Med Assoc* 1999; **281**: 908–913.

33. Bridges CB, Thompson WW, Meltzer MI *et al.* Effectiveness and cost-benefit of influenza vaccination of healthy working adults: a randomized controlled trial. *J Am Med Assoc* 2000; **284**: 1655–1663.

34. Nichol KL, Lind A, Margolis KL *et al.* The effectiveness of

vaccination against influenza in healthy, working adults. *New Engl J Med* 1995; **333**: 889–893.

35. Nichol KL, Mallon KP, Mendelman PM. Cost benefit of influenza vaccination in healthy, working adults: an economic analysis based on the results of a clinical trial of trivalent live attenuated influenza virus vaccine. *Vaccine* 2003; **21**: 2207–2217.

36. Campbell DS, Rumley MH. Cost-effectiveness of the influenza vaccine in a healthy, working-age population. *J Occup Environ Med* 1997; **5**: 408–414.

37. Office of Technology Assessment. Cost-effectiveness of influenza vaccination. Washington, DC: Congress of the United States, 1981.

38. Centers for Disease Control and Prevention. Prevention and control of influenza. Recommendations of the Advisory Committee on Immunization Practices (ACIP). MMWR 2002; **51**(RR-3).

39. Neuzil KM, Dupont WD, Wright PF, Edwards KM. Efficacy of inactivated and cold-adapted vaccines against influenza A infection, 1985 to 1990: the pediatric experience. *Pediatr Infect Dis J* 2001; **20**: 733–740.

40. Neuzil KM, Edwards KM. Influenza vaccines in children. *Semin Pediatr Infect Dis* 2002; **13**: 174–181.

41. Heikkinen T, Ruuskanen O, Waris M *et al*. Influenza vaccination in the prevention of acute otitis media in children. *Am J Dis Child* 1991; **145**: 445–448.

42. Monto AS, Davenport FM, Napier JA, Francis T. Modification of an outbreak of influenza in Tecumseh, Michigan by vaccination of schoolchildren. *J Infect Dis* 1970; **122**: 16–25.

43. Reichert TA, Sugaya N, Fedson DS *et al*. The Japanese experience with vaccinating schoolchildren against influenza. *New Engl J Med* 2001; **344**: 889–896.

44. Cohen GM, Nettleman MD. Economic impact of influenza

vaccination in preschool children. *Pediatrics* 2000; **106**:973–976.

45. Park CL, Frank AL, Sullivan M, Jindal P, Baxter BD. Influenza vaccination of children during acute asthma exacerbation and concurrent prednisone therapy. *Pediatrics* 1996; **98**: 196–200.

46. Safranek TJ, Lawrence DN, Kurland LT *et al.* Reassessment of the association between Guillain–Barré syndrome and receipt of swine influenza vaccine in 1976–1977: results of a two-state study. *Am J Epidemiol* 1991; **133**: 940–951.

47. Lasky T, Terracciano GJ, Magder L, *et al.* The Guillain-Barré syndrome and the 1992–1993 and 1993–1994 influenza vaccines. *New Engl J Med* 1998; **339**: 1797–1802.

Treatment and Prophylaxis with Antivirals

Influenza often presents to the primary-care physician several days into an illness that begins with fever, myalgias and cough. Patients, on their own or at the recommendation of their physician, may use paracetamol, aspirin or other non-steroidal anti-inflammatory medications for symptomatic relief. The symptoms of influenza might be regarded by the patient as a bacterial infection and the reason for a visit to the physician is often to obtain a prescription for antibiotics. This, and/or inaccurate diagnosis of the disease (see pp. 86–106), may lead to over-prescribing of antibiotics for uncomplicated influenza illness, which contributes to the development of microbial resistance to antibiotics. Bacterial complications of influenza generally present 5–7 days after the onset of illness and during a phase of apparent recovery and then recurrence of symptoms.

Clearly, vaccination, as discussed in the previous chapter, remains the method of choice for influenza prophylaxis. However, under specific conditions – for example, when vaccination has not been performed or cannot be performed, perhaps because of hypersensitivity to egg proteins, or when vaccinated subjects are not fully protected – the use of specific antiviral drugs should be considered for treatment or prevention of influenza infection. Antiviral drugs effective against influenza include the M2 channel inhibitors amantadine (Symmetrel, Lysovir, Symadine) and rimantadine (Flumadine), and the neuraminidase inhibitors zanamivir (Relenza) and oseltamivir (Tamiflu). These drugs interfere with specific steps in the replication cycle of influenza virus, either at the level of virus entry or at the level of virus assembly release from the infected cell.

The use of M2 channel inhibitors, which are active only against influenza A viruses, has been limited by the occurrence of adverse side-effects and the risk of induction of drug-resistant viral strains. The neuraminidase inhibitors represent a novel class of anti-influenza drugs that are active against both influenza A and B viruses; adverse effects are very limited and, thus far, significant development of resistant viral variants has not been reported for these drugs.

Key Messages

- Antibiotics are often inappropriately prescribed in cases of influenza-like illness where uncomplicated influenza infection presents to the physician.
- Antiviral drugs must be initiated within 24–48 hours of the onset of symptoms for the treatment of influenza.
- The use of M2 inhibitors has been limited by the induction of drug-resistant strains of influenza.
- Particularly in older people, the use of M2 inhibitors has been limited by their adverse effects and need for dose adjustment due to renal excretion of the drugs.
- Antiviral drugs must be taken daily through the period of exposure risk for effective prophylaxis against influenza.
- Data on the benefits of neuraminidase inhibitors among high-risk populations are limited.
- Thus far there are few observations of induction of drug-resistant influenza strains by neuraminidase inhibitors.
- In contrast to the M2 inhibitors, neuraminidase inhibitors do not need dose adjustment to reduce side-effects.
- In the initial phase of an influenza pandemic, antivirals will be the only means to combat its impact.

Mechanisms of action of antivirals

Amantadine and rimantadine were the first generation of influenza antiviral agents.[1] These compounds specifically block the ion channel function of the M2 protein of influenza A virus (see pp. 23–44), thus interfering with corresponding specific steps in the viral life cycle. The neuraminidase inhibitors are novel drugs, designed on the basis of the three-dimensional structure of the influenza

A and B neuraminidase[2] (see pp. 23–44). The mechanisms of action of the four available specific anti-influenza viral drugs are summarized in Figure 28.

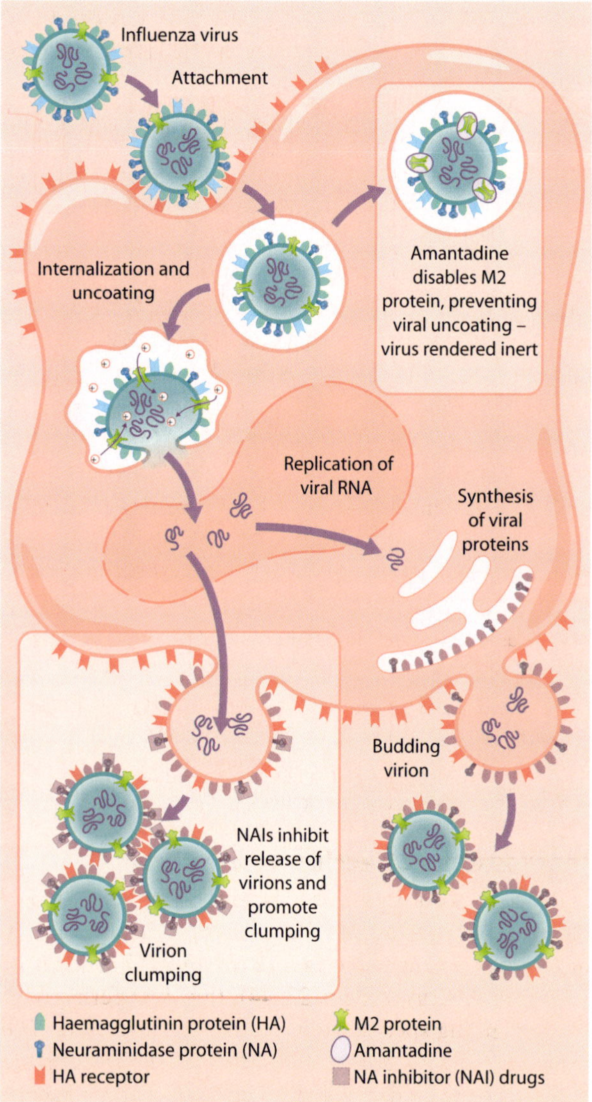

The M2 channel inhibitors – amantadine and rimantadine

At high concentrations (>15 μg/ml), amantadine and rimantadine non-specifically raise the pH within cellular endosomes, thus inhibiting or retarding the acid-induced conformational change in the viral HA. However, the required concentrations of the drugs are not generally attained *in vivo*. At low, pharmacologically relevant concentrations (<0.75 μg/ml), amantadine and rimantadine specifically inhibit the ion channel activity of the M2 protein, probably through direct binding to the pore region of the protein.[3] In doing so, the drugs inhibit acidification of the interior of susceptible viruses and dissociation of the M1 protein from the viral nucleocapsid (Figure 28), which is a necessary step in uncoating of the viral genome during infection (see pp. 23–44). In addition, M2 protects HA against premature exposure to low pH, while HA is in transit to the plasma membrane of infected cells, by temporarily neutralizing the low pH of the trans-Golgi network.[4] Amantadine and rimantadine counteract this protection and thus indirectly induce a premature conformational change in HA, inactivating the protein (Figure 28). Since M2 is present only in influenza A viruses, amantadine and rimantadine are active only against influenza A.

Figure 28. The mechanism by which antiviral drugs interrupt the replicative cycle of influenza is illustrated. M2 inhibitors prevent the M2-mediated acidification of the interior of the virus while it resides in endosomes and the subsequent uncoating of the viral genome, thus inhibiting viral replication. Neuraminidase inhibitors (NAIs) prevent cleavage of sialic acid residues and thus newly formed virus cannot be released from the cell surface to infect adjacent cells; also, virus particles remain associated to one another. "The treatment of influenza with antiviral drugs". Reprinted from *CMAJ* 07-Jan-03; **168(1)**: 49–57 by permission of the publisher.

The neuraminidase inhibitors – zanamivir and oseltamivir

Influenza A and B viruses (but not influenza C viruses) possess neuraminidase on their outer surface, an enzyme essential for release of virus from infected cells, for prevention of formation of viral aggregates and for viral spread within the respiratory tract.[2] Neuraminidase cleaves the receptor for influenza A and B viruses, sialic acid, from glycoproteins and glycolipids. Zanamivir and oseltamivir are analogues of sialic acid, as shown in Figure 29.[2] These compounds specifically inhibit all nine neuraminidase subtypes in nature, including the subtypes contained in the avian strains of influenza A H5N1 and H9N2 that have infected humans.

The inhibition of neuraminidase on both influenza A and B viruses has two important consequences.[2] First, it hinders the passage of the virus through the mucus of the respiratory tract and thus retards initial infection of epithelial cells. Second, it inhibits the release of new viral particles from the surface of infected cells and thus retards spreading of the virus through the respiratory tract of the host.

Antivirals in treatment and prophylaxis of influenza

Table 19 presents a comparison between the different antiviral drugs available for treatment (amantadine, rimantadine and oseltamivir) and prophylaxis (amantadine, rimantadine, oseltamivir and zanamivir) of influenza. Only oseltamivir and zanamivir are effective against influenza B. The UK National Institute for Clinical Excellence no longer approves the use of amantadine for treatment of influenza,[5] the reasons for which will be discussed below.

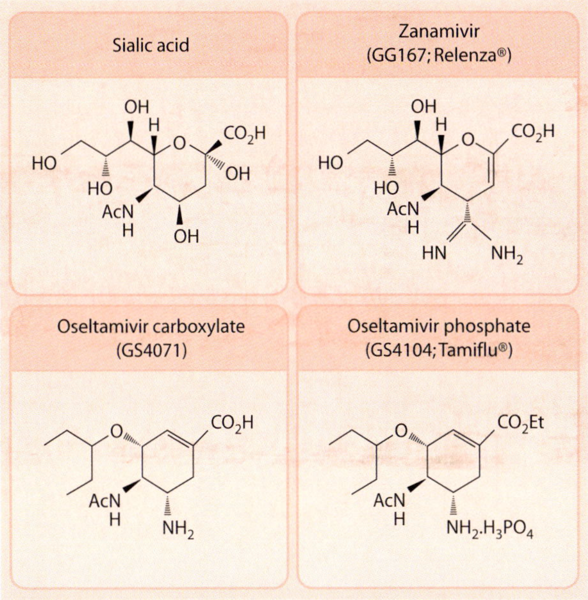

Figure 29. The neuraminidase inhibitors zanamivir and oseltamivir are structural analogs of sialic acid, which is the substrate of neuraminidase (NA) and the receptor for the influenza virus HA. Zanamivir and oseltamivir bind to the substrate binding site of NA, thus blocking its enzymatic activity. Zanamivir (GG167 or Relenza®) is inhaled or administered intranasally. Oseltamivir is given as the oral prodrug oseltamivir phosphate (GS4104 or Tamiflu®), which is converted in the liver to oseltamivir carboxylate GS4071, the active drug.

The influenza antiviral drugs should only be used to treat patients if the clinical picture meets the criteria for influenza-like illness and if influenza activity has been reported in the area. Table 20 lists indications for antiviral drugs against influenza.

Comparison of antiviral drugs for prophylaxis and treatment of influenza

Drug	Trade name	Influenza type	Dosing for prophylaxis	Dosing for treatment	Main side-effects
Amantadine	Symmetrel®	A	Age 1–9 years: 5 mg/kg/day, p.o. div b.i.d. Age 9 and up: 100 mg p.o. b.i.d.	Age 1–9 years: 5 mg/kg/day, p.o. div b.i.d. Age 9 and up: 100 mg p.o. b.i.d.	Central nervous system
Rimantadine	Flumadine®	A	Age 1–10 years: 5 mg/kg/day, p.o. q.d. Age 10 and up: 100 mg p.o. b.i.d.	Adults: 100 mg p.o. b.i.d.	Central nervous system
Zanamivir	Relenza®	A and B	N/A	Age >7 years: 10 mg inhaled b.i.d.	Bronchial
Oseltamivir	Tamiflu®	A and B	Age ≥ 13 years: 75 mg p.o. q.d.	Age 1–12 years: dose per weight Age 13 and up: 75 mg p.o. b.i.d.	Gastrointestinal

*For children who weigh <15 kg the dose is 30 mg b.i.d.; for those who weigh 15–23 kg, it is 45 mg b.i.d.; for those who weigh 23–40 kg, it is 60 mg b.i.d.; and for those who weigh >40 kg, it is 75 mg b.i.d.

Table 19. Comparison of antiviral drugs for prophylaxis and treatment of influenza. Reproduced from La Rosa AM and Whimbey E. Respiratory viruses. In: Cohen J, Powderly WG, editors. *Infectious Diseases*, 2nd edn, 2003 with permission from Elsevier.

Indications for antiviral drugs against influenza
• Patients at risk and their household contacts, who have not (yet) been vaccinated at the time when influenza infections are becoming widespread in an area.
• Control of an outbreak in a (semi-)closed community (e.g. nursing home).
• Patients at risk with a known hypersensitivity to chicken proteins (contraindication for vaccination).
• Vaccine mismatch between vaccine component and circulating virus strain.
• Pandemic threat with no vaccine (yet) available.

Table 20. Indications for antiviral drugs against influenza. Adapted from CDC, Prevention and control of influenza. Recommendations ACIP. *MMWR Recomm Rep* 2004: **53**(RR-6): 1–40.

Treatment of influenza

All influenza antiviral agents have to be administered within 24–48 hours of disease onset. The drugs are given orally, except for zanamivir, which is inhaled. Influenza antiviral drugs diminish the severity of clinical symptoms and shorten the duration of uncomplicated influenza disease by an average of 1 day (from about 7 to 6 days). To reduce the risk of drug resistance (see below), amantadine or rimantadine should be discontinued as soon as clinically appropriate, usually after 3–5 days or within 24–48 hours after the disappearance of symptoms. For zanamivir and oseltamivir, the recommended duration of treatment is 5 days.

Evidence for the effectiveness of these four antiviral agents is based primarily on studies of uncomplicated influenza in adults.[6] None of the drugs has been shown to prevent serious complications, such as pneumonia or the exacerbation of underlying disease. Data are limited regarding their effectiveness in the treatment of influenza among people at high risk of serious complications and among paediatric populations.

Both M2 channel blockers interact with a variety of different medicines, which can exacerbate their toxicity, including antihistamines, anticholinergics, co-trimoxazole, triamterene, quinine, quinidine, monoamine oxidase inhibitors, cimetidine, aspirin and paracetamol. When drugs such as antihistamines, antidepressants or minor tranquillizers are co-administered, patients should be monitored closely for CNS side-effects.

Adverse effects

The most common side-effects of the M2 inhibitors are CNS complaints (anxiety, difficulty concentrating, insomnia, dizziness, headache and jitteriness) and gastrointestinal upset. While the CNS complaints are minor in younger adults, these symptoms may be very prominent in older adults, particularly with the use of amantadine. Reduction of these symptoms depends on dose adjustments based on creatinine clearance. Patients who receive amantadine may develop antimuscarinic effects, orthostatic hypotension and congestive heart failure. Particularly in the elderly or those with renal failure, serious CNS side-effects due to amantadine (and less often rimantadine) include confusion, disorientation, mood alterations, memory disturbances, delusions, nightmares, ataxia, tremors, seizures, coma, acute psychosis, slurred speech, visual disturbances, delirium, oculogyric episodes and hallucinations.[1] Amantadine causes CNS side-effects in about 15–30% of people, as well as dose-related abnormalities in psychomotor testing. Amantadine (and possibly rimantadine) may increase the risk of seizures in those with a history of seizures.

In general, neuraminidase inhibitors have fewer adverse effects than the M2 channel blockers. Oseltamivir is normally well tolerated but may induce gastrointestinal side-effects, including nausea and vomiting, especially if the drug is not taken with food. Other infrequent possible adverse events include insomnia, vertigo and fever. Postmarketing reports suggest that oseltamivir may be associated rarely with skin rash, hepatic dysfunction or thrombocytopenia.

The inhaled zanamivir may induce bronchospasm (potentially severe) in those with underlying lung disease. Current guidelines advise against the use of zanamivir in patients with hyperreactive airways, unless the patient is closely monitored and has a fast-acting inhaled bronchodilator available when inhaling zanamivir.[7] Other less frequent side-effects include diarrhoea, nausea, headache and dizziness. Zanamivir is associated with low bioavailability and no clinically significant drug interactions have been recognized.

Influenza prophylaxis with antivirals

Under specific conditions as indicated above, influenza antivirals may be used for prevention of influenza infection. Both of the M2 blockers are 70–90% effective in preventing illness from influenza A infection in healthy adults.[8] When used as prophylaxis, they permit subclinical infection (whilst preventing illness) and allow development of protective antibodies. Both drugs have been studied extensively as a component of influenza outbreak-control programmes and can limit the spread of influenza in nursing homes,[9] as discussed below.

Despite the fact that, of the neuraminidase inhibitors, only oseltamivir has been approved for prophylaxis, both drugs have been shown to be similarly effective (82–84%) in preventing influenza in community studies of healthy adults.[10,11] Fewer data are available regarding their prophylactic use in closed settings or among patients with chronic medical conditions compared to the M2 blockers, but one study with oseltamivir reported a 92% reduction in influenza illness among nursing home residents.[12]

There are no data regarding prophylactic efficacy of any of the four antiviral agents among people with severe immunosuppression. In such people, prophylaxis can be considered for those expected to have an inadequate antibody response to influenza vaccine, including HIV-positive individuals, and in particular those with advanced disease. Such patients should be monitored closely for interactions with other drugs used to treat HIV-positive individuals.

For the purposes of prevention, after an outbreak has been reported, vulnerable adults can be vaccinated and simultaneously receive prophylactic treatment for 2–3 weeks until sufficient antibodies have been generated by vaccination.[13,14] In individuals who remain unvaccinated, the drug must be taken each day for the duration of influenza activity in the community to be maximally effective as prophylaxis. Children under 9 years old receiving the influenza vaccine for the first time can require 6 weeks of prophylaxis (i.e. for 4 weeks after the first dose of vaccine and an additional 2 weeks after the second).

Development of drug resistance

Resistance to amantadine and rimantadine occurs as a result of amino acid substitutions in the transmembrane portion of the M2 protein. Although resistant wild-type virus is uncommon (<1%),[15] resistant viruses may rapidly emerge within 2–4 days after the start of therapy in up to 30% of patients.[16] Emergence of resistant virus does not appear to cause a rebound in illness in immunocompetent adults, but may be associated with protracted illness and shedding in immunocompromised hosts.[17] Importantly, resistant virus can be spread to others and has caused failures of antiviral prophylaxis under close contact conditions, as in nursing homes and households.[1] The resistant viruses appear to retain wild-type pathogenicity and cause an influenza illness indistinguishable from that caused by susceptible strains.

The use of neuraminidase inhibitors to date for both prophylaxis and treatment has not been associated with clinically relevant development of antiviral resistance. This often makes them, despite the fact that they are expensive, the preferred drugs relative to the low-cost amantadine and rimantadine, but ultimately cost considerations may also influence the choice of the drug that is used.

Control of influenza outbreaks in (semi-)closed settings

In closed institutions the use of antiviral drugs both for treatment and prophylaxis is a key component in the control of influenza outbreaks. When an outbreak occurs in a nursing home, all residents should receive prophylaxis, whether or not they have been vaccinated. This should continue for a minimum of 2 weeks and until approximately 1 week after the last case has been identified. Prophylaxis should be considered for all unvaccinated staff, and, in the case of outbreaks caused by a variant strain not well matched by the vaccine, prophylaxis should be considered for all employees, both vaccinated and unvaccinated. Dose of drug should be determined on an individual basis.[18]

Prevention can also be considered for controlling outbreaks in other (semi-)closed settings (e.g. dormitories, schools, cruise ships).

Antivirals and pandemic preparedness

The anticipated problems of induction of resistance to the M2 inhibitors would quickly diminish the efficacy of this class of antiviral drugs in the early management of pandemic influenza, i.e. when a vaccine is still unavailable. Thus, the advent of the neuraminidase inhibitors has been a welcome alternative to prevention and treatment in this situation. However, a number of issues related to the use of the neuraminidase inhibitors remain to be addressed. The half-life and cost of these medications and their unproven efficacy in high-risk populations (potentially in the absence of a pandemic vaccine) remain significant barriers to their inclusion in pandemic planning strategies. The need for large stockpiles of lower cost, more efficacious and easily administered medications has been identified.[19] Co-ordinated public health planning and the commitment of government to the development of a realistic plan for including antivirals in pandemic planning are necessary.[18]

References

1. Hayden FG, Aoki FY. Amantadine, rimantadine, and related agents. In: Barriere SL, editor. *Antimicrobial Therapy and Vaccines*. Baltimore: Williams & Wilkins; 1999; pp. 1344–1365.

2. Colman PM. Influenza virus neuraminidase: structure, antibodies, and inhibitors. *Protein Sci* 1994; **3**: 1687–1696.

3. Wang C, Takeuchi K, Pinto LH, Lamb RA. Ion channel activity of influenza A virus M2 protein: characterization of the amantadine block. *J Virol* 1993; **67**: 5585–5594.

4. Ruigrok RW, Hirst EM, Hay AJ. The specific inhibition of influenza A virus maturation by amantadine: an electron microscopic examination. *J Gen Virol* 1991; **72**: 191–194.

5. National Institute for Clinical Excellence. Guidance on the use of zanamivir, oseltamivir and amantadine for the treatment of influenza. In: *Flu – zanamivir (review), amantadine and oseltamivir*. 2003; **58**. http://www.nice.org.uk.

6. Food and Drug Administration. Subject: safe and appropriate use of influenza drugs [Public Health Advisory]. Rockville, MD: US Department of Health and Human Services, Food and Drug Administration, 2000.

7. Prevention and control of influenza: Recommendations of the Advisory Committee on Immunization Practices (ACIP). *MMWR Morb Mortal Wkly Rep* 2002; **51**: 1.

8. Demicheli V, Jefferson T, Rivetti D, Deeks J. Prevention and early treatment of influenza in healthy adults. *Vaccine* 2000; **18**: 957–1003.

9. Nicholson KG. Use of antivirals in influenza in the elderly: prophylaxis and therapy. *Gerontology* 1996; **42**: 280–289.

10. Monto AS, Pichichero ME, Blanckenberg SJ *et al.* Zanamivir prophylaxis: an effective strategy for the prevention of influenza types A and B within households. *J Infect Dis* 2002; **186**: 1582–1588.

11. Hayden FG, Atmar RL, Schilling M *et al.* Use of the selective oral neuraminidase inhibitor oseltamivir to prevent influenza. *New Engl J Med* 1999; **341**: 1336–1343.

12. Peters PH Jr, Gravenstein S, Norwood P *et al.* Long-term use of oseltamivir for the prophylaxis of influenza in a vaccinated frail older population. *J Am Geriatr Soc* 2001; **49**: 1025–1031.

13. Gross PA, Russo C, Dran S, Cataruozolo P, Munk G, Lancey SC. Time to earliest peak serum antibody response to influenza vaccine in the elderly. *Clin Diagn Lab Immunol* 1997; **4**: 491–492.

14. Brokstad KA, Cox RJ, Olofsson J, Jonsson R, Haaheim LR. Parenteral influenza vaccination induces a rapid systemic and local immune response. *J Infect Dis* 1995; **171**: 198–203.

15. Ziegler T, Hemphill ML, Ziegler ML *et al.* Low incidence of rimantadine resistance in field isolates of influenza A viruses. *J Infect Dis* 1999; **180**: 935–939.

16. Hayden FG. Amantadine and rimantadine: clinical aspects. In: Richman DD, editor. *Antiviral Drug Resistance*. New York: Wiley; 1996.

17. Englund JA, Champlin RE, Wyde PR *et al.* Common emergence of amantadine- and rimantadine-resistant influenza A viruses in symptomatic immunocompromised adults. *Clin Infect Dis* 1998; **26**:1418–1424.

18. Monto AS. The role of antivirals in the control of influenza. *Vaccine* 2003;**21**:1796–1800.

19. Stohr K. Preventing and treating influenza. *Br Med J* 2003; **326**: 1223–1224.

Novel Developments in the Control of Influenza

Current inactivated influenza vaccines significantly reduce influenza morbidity and mortality among at-risk populations (see pp. 9–22 and pp. 124–151). Furthermore, these vaccines have an excellent safety record. However, there remain limitations. First, the efficacy of inactivated vaccines, particularly in the elderly, is lower than that of many other prophylactic viral vaccines. Also, current vaccine formulations are probably not efficacious enough to induce adequate protection against entirely new pandemic virus subtypes that might enter the population. Second, the current route of vaccine administration by intramuscular injection often represents a barrier for acceptance of the vaccine. Third, vaccine virus growth in chicken embryos poses limitations to the flexibility of the production process, particularly under conditions of a sudden high demand for vaccine, such as in the case of an emerging pandemic.

It is clear, therefore, that there is a need for novel influenza vaccine modalities, not only for improvement of the clinical effectiveness of flu vaccination in current target groups, but also for optimizing pandemic preparedness.[1–5] In addition, there is a great deal of interest in vaccine formulations that may be delivered via routes other than injection – for example, locally with a nasal spray. Various novel influenza vaccine modalities, as well as new approaches for vaccine virus production, will be discussed below. Finally, options for an improved vaccination coverage and avenues towards universal flu vaccination will be considered.

Key Messages

- Although current inactivated influenza vaccines have been shown to subtantially reduce influenza morbidity and mortality, there remains a need for novel influenza vaccines with improved efficacy, particularly among the elderly.
- More efficacious influenza vaccines are also needed for an improved influenza pandemic preparedness.
- Novel vaccine modalities for the elderly should induce not only a robust antibody response, but also T-cell-mediated immunity.
- There is a need for influenza vaccines that may be administered by routes other than injection, since injection sometimes represents a barrier for acceptance of the vaccine.
- Vaccines administered intranasally would have the additional advantage of inducing local immunity in the respiratory tract.
- Along with egg-based vaccine production, growth of vaccine virus on cell-culture substrates will considerably improve vaccine supply capabilities, which is of particular importance under conditions of pandemic threat.
- Primary-care physicians are in a key position to help improve the use of available influenza vaccines.

Novel inactivated influenza vaccines with improved efficacy

One of the limitations of current inactivated influenza vaccines is their suboptimal efficacy among the elderly,[6–8] which appears to be primarily related to a diminishing T-cell activity with age (see pp. 68–85).[9] These age-related changes in cell-mediated immunity put specific demands on novel vaccine modalities. The presentation form of conventional vaccines is not optimal for stimulation of cell-mediated immunity, particularly cytotoxic T lymphocyte (CTL) activity. Moreover, as opposed to the viral HA that directs the antibody response against influenza, the antigenic determinants of CTL activity are primarily derived from the internal proteins of the virus (see pp. 68–85).

It is for these reasons that, particularly in the case of new vaccines for the elderly, improvements of the formulations are sought at the level of T-cell immunity, in addition to induction of antibody responses. Accordingly, antibody titres are unlikely to remain the sole reliable correlate of protection. In evaluating the efficacy of novel generations of flu vaccines, it will therefore be necessary to consider, besides antibody titres, also other parameters, including T-cell-mediated immunity.

Current inactivated vaccines exhibit relatively poor immunogenicity in immunologically naive individuals, such as small children, who have not had prior exposure to virus or vaccine.[10] Likewise, in the case of a pandemic outbreak, current vaccine formulations are unlikely to provide adequate protection, again as a result of a total lack of pre-exposure of the population to the emerging new virus subtype.[11] More powerful vaccines are needed which, in these cases, primarily need to induce a very robust antibody response against HA.

Adjuvanted vaccines

The use of adjuvants represents one way to improve the efficacy of vaccines. An adjuvanted influenza vaccine, FluAD®, has recently been licensed in Europe. It is formulated as an oil-in-water emulsion, referred to as MF59, containing squalene, Tween 80 and sorbitan trioleate. Although this vaccine, which contains the usual 15 μg of HA per strain, had an only modest immunopotentiating effect in primed individuals, including the elderly,[12] it has a clear-cut advantage over non-adjuvanted vaccine in immunologically naive individuals. In a recent study among volunteers, involving an experimental MF59-adjuvanted vaccine against the H5N1 virus, significantly higher rates of seroconversion were achieved with the adjuvanted vaccine as compared to the non-adjuvanted vaccine.[11] On the other hand, the MF59-

adjuvanted vaccine appears to be more reactogenic than non-adjuvanted vaccine.[12]

A promising class of adjuvants is derived from bacterial enterotoxins, such as cholera toxin (CT) and the *E. coli* heat-labile enterotoxin (LT).[13] These molecules, including a number of detoxified CT or LT variants, are of particular interest in the context of mucosal vaccine delivery and potentiation of local secretory IgA responses, as discussed in more detail below. However, the non-toxic recombinant B subunit of LT (LTB) also had potent adjuvant activity when administered intramuscularly to mice along with influenza subunit vaccine.[14]

Immune stimulation can also be induced by the use of specific cytokines, including IL-2 and GM-CSF. In murine preclinical studies, these cytokine adjuvants strongly promoted antibody responses to influenza surface glycoproteins, including neuraminidase, in a liposome formulation, mediating cross-reactive protection against a variety of influenza A strains.[15] A similar experimental vaccine has recently been evaluated in human clinical trials.[16] Stringent safety testing seems mandatory, since cytokines may well have multiple biological effects besides adjuvant activity.

Adjuvants may also reduce the current requirement for a dosing of 15 μg of HA per strain. This is of particular importance in the context of vaccine development for future pandemics, where no doubt the demand for vaccine will be higher than the available supplies. In a volunteer study, involving whole-inactivated H9N2 or H2N2 vaccine supplemented with alum adjuvant, a two- to eight-fold reduced amount of HA per dose sufficed for induction of antibody levels similar to those induced by 15 μg of unadjuvanted whole-virus vaccine.[17]

Virosomes as a novel vaccine presentation system

Another approach by which the response to inactivated viral vaccines can be improved, involves modification of the way in which the antigen is presented to the immune system. Virosomes are a presentation form that closely mimics the native virus. Virosomes are virus-like particles lacking the genetic material of the native virus. They are generated by a reconstitution procedure,[18,19] involving treatment of influenza virus with an appropriate detergent such that the viral envelope is selectively solubilized, leaving the nucleocapsid surrounded by the M1 protein intact. After separation of the nucleocapsid fraction by ultracentrifugation, the detergent is removed from the supernatant in a controlled fashion such that viral envelopes ("virosomes") are reformed. Figure 30 shows a schematic representation and an electron micrograph of influenza virosomes.

Functionally reconstituted virosomes preserve the receptor-binding and membrane fusion activity of the viral HA. This implies that these virosomes, like the native virus, are internalized by cells through receptor-mediated endocytosis and fusion from within acidic endosomes (see pp. 23–44). However, since the virosomes are empty vesicles, lacking the genetic material of the virus, this does not result in infection of the cells. Through fusion of the virosomes with the endosomal membrane, a continuity is established between the virosomal lumen and the cell cytosol, while the HA is introduced into the endosomal membrane.

During the preparation of virosomes, biologically active molecules, including protein antigens, may be encapsulated in the virosomal lumen. Fusion of the virosomes from within the endosomal cell compartment will result in delivery of these virosome-encapsulated compounds to the target cell cytosol.[19] Accordingly, interaction of fusion-active virosomes with antigen-presenting cells (APCs), such as dendritic cells (DCs), results in delivery of virosome-encapsulated protein antigen to the lumen of the cells. In this manner, the antigen gains access to the MHC class I presentation pathway[20] (Figure 31). In addition, interaction of virosomes with DCs results in activation and maturation of DCs.[20] *In vivo* studies in mice have demonstrated that fusion-active virosomes, containing an encapsulated protein antigen, efficiently prime

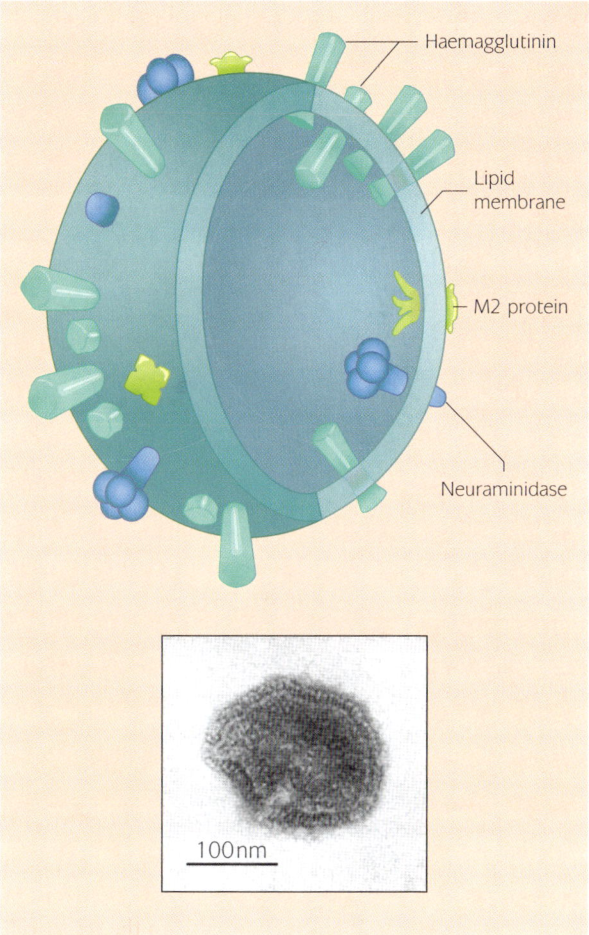

Figure 30. (Top) Model of a virosome derived from influenza virus. (Bottom) Electron micrograph of a virosome. Image courtesy of Laura Bungener, University of Groningen, Groningen, The Netherlands.

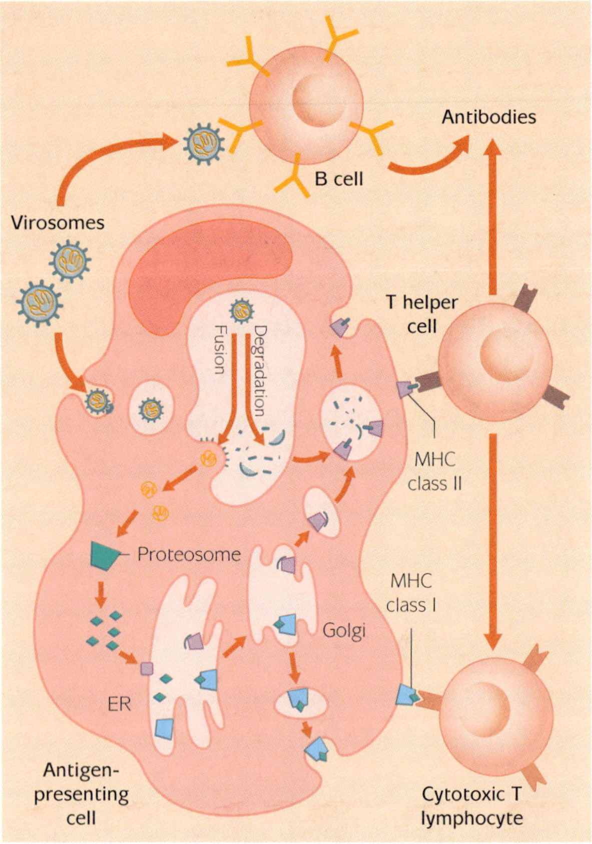

Figure 31. Interaction of virosomes with cells of the immune system. By virtue of the repetititve arrangement of HA on the virosome surface, virosomes interact efficiently with immunoglobulin receptors on B lymphocytes. Virosomes are also taken up avidly by antigen-presenting cells, particularly dendritic cells. Antigens on the virosome surface, as well as antigens derived from degraded virosomes, enter the MHC class II pathway, activating T helper cells. Antigens inside the virosomes, through fusion of the virosomes, access the cytosolic MHC class I presentation pathway, activating cytotoxic T lymphocytes. Adapted from Huckriede A *et al*. Influenza virosomes: combining optimal presentation of hemagglutinin with immunopotentiating activity. *Vaccine* 2003; **21**: 925–931[21] with permission from Elsevier.

a class I MHC-restricted CTL response against the encapsulated antigen.[21] In addition, virosomes induce a potent antibody response against the virosomal HA. Thus, virosomes induce a broad immune response, priming both the humoral and cellular arms of the immune system.[21,22]

Currently, there is a virosome-based influenza vaccine, Inflexal V®, on the market. Another virosomal influenza vaccine, Invivac®, has been registered in Europe.[23] Like Inflexal V®, this vaccine has an excellent safety and immunogenicity profile.[23]

Immune-stimulating complexes

Immune-stimulating complexes, or ISCOMs, represent another presentation form for membrane-associated antigens. ISCOMs are cage-like structures (Figure 32) that are formed from phospholipids, cholesterol and saponins, the latter functioning not only as an essential component of the ISCOM structure, but also as a built-in adjuvant.[24]

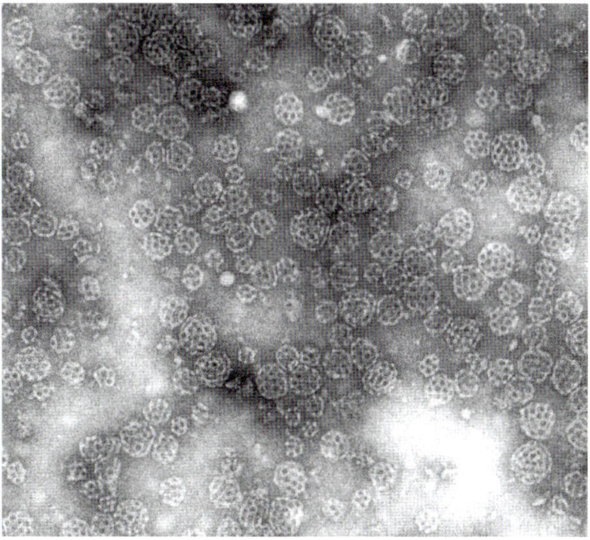

Figure 32. Electron micrograph of immune-stimulating complexes (ISCOMs). Image courtesy of Guus Rimmelzwaan, Erasmus MC, Rotterdam, The Netherlands.

Integral membrane proteins, such as influenza HA, may be incorporated in the ISCOM structure during their preparation. ISCOMs have been shown to strongly promote antibody responses to incorporated protein antigens in a number of preclinical animal models, including a non-human primate model.[25] Also, ISCOMs have the capacity to introduce antigens into the MHC class I presentation pathway, thus inducing CD8-positive CTL activity.[26] An ISCOM-based influenza vaccine for horses is on the market. In a human influenza vaccine trial, however, ISCOMs did not show enhanced antibody responses as compared to conventional inactivated influenza vaccines.[27] In addition, there remains an issue with regard to the reactogenicity of the vaccine due to the presence of the saponin component in the ISCOM structure.

Other approaches

Several experimental approaches for the development of novel, more effective, influenza vaccine modalities are under investigation. These include approaches involving DNA immunization[28,29] and experimental vaccines targeted at conserved viral antigens such as M2 and/or NP, with the purpose of inducing an immune response that would be cross-reactive to different influenza drift variants or even subtypes.

DNA immunization relies on the *in situ* synthesis of protein antigens after intramuscular administration of naked DNA. As protein antigens may also be synthesized within APCs, DNA immunization is expected to access the MHC class I presentation pathway and thus may stimulate CTL activity. DNA immunization against a number of influenza antigens, including HA and NP, has given promising results in murine model systems, but appears less effective in humans. In addition, safety concerns remain with regard to the use of DNA for mass vaccination purposes.

Very promising results have been obtained with the use of an experimental M2-based vaccine in mice.[30] However, a more recent study in pigs has raised considerable concern, in that animals vaccinated with an experimental M2/NP DNA vaccine exhibited exacerbation of disease upon challenge, rather than protection.[31] Clearly, more data are needed to determine whether M2 represents an appropriate antigen for use in novel flu vaccine modalities.

Mucosal delivery of influenza vaccines

To those of us fearing needles, the current mode of vaccine administration by injection may represent a barrier for taking an annual flu shot. In addition, administration of the vaccine by intramuscular injection is not in line with the site of entry of the influenza virus via mucosal surfaces of the nasal cavity, and does not generally induce a local mucosal secretory IgA (sIgA) response as the first line of defence against incoming virus. It is for these reasons that there is considerable interest in mucosal influenza vaccine formulations.

A major hurdle in the development of such vaccines has been the comparatively low immunogenicity of inactivated vaccine formulations upon intranasal delivery, especially when induction of serum HI antibodies is taken as the marker of vaccine efficacy. It appears that mucosal delivery of inactivated vaccines is not a very efficient way of inducing antibody responses,[32] and that stimulation of the mucosal immune system requires the use of an adjuvant. Alternatively, live attenuated virus preparations may be used, such as cold-adapted viruses that only replicate in the upper respiratory tract, inducing both local and systemic antibody responses as well as cellular immunity.

Adjuvanted inactivated intranasal vaccines

A number of candidate adjuvanted inactivated influenza vaccines for intranasal administration are under development. These include a subunit vaccine formulated in MF59,[33] and a proteosome vaccine, FluInsure™, containing outer membrane proteins of *Neisseria meningitidis*.[34] In clinical studies, these vaccines have been shown to induce high levels of serum HI antibodies and a local sIgA response in the nasal cavity. The FluInsure™ vaccine has recently been evaluated in a large-scale placebo-controlled field efficacy study, enrolling 1349 healthy subjects aged 18 to 64. The study was conducted in the 2003-2004 influenza season, under conditions of a suboptimal match between the vaccine composition and the circulating A/Fujian-like (H3N2) virus. Yet, the FluInsure™ vaccine, in a single-dose regimen, showed a high 67% efficacy in preventing influenza-like illness.

Another intranasal influenza vaccine, NasalFlu®, containing native, non-detoxified, *E. coli* heat-labile enterotoxin (LT) as an adjuvant, was licensed in Switzerland in 2001. However, soon after it was introduced, the vaccine had to be withdrawn, because of an increased number of cases of Bell's palsy in association with the vaccination.[35] Although not formally established, it is likely that the occurrence of this complication is due to the toxic activity of the unmodified *E. coli* LT, the intranasal administration of the vaccine possibly allowing migration of the toxin to the brain. In view of this complication, the use of detoxified variants of CT and LT would appear to be preferable. Non-toxic recombinant LTB retained potent adjuvant activity when administered intranasally to mice together with influenza subunit vaccine, inducing high levels of systemic IgG and local sIgA. The mice were completely protected from infection upon viral challenge.[14]

Live attenuated vaccines

An alternative approach for intranasal vaccination involves the use of a live attenuated influenza vaccine (LAIV). Intranasally delivered LAIVs more closely mimic a natural infection than do injected inactivated vaccines. LAIV vaccines have been used for decades in Russia,[36] but unfortunately not much information about their safety and efficacy is available. In the 1960s, a research programme was initiated in the USA to develop LAIVs.[37] This programme led to the FDA approval of FluMist® in the USA in 2003 for individuals between ages 5 and 49 years.

LAIVs are made by reassortment of a temperature-sensitive, cold-adapted (*ca*) parent virus and an actual vaccine virus strain. The *ca* virus replicates at the reduced temperatures of the upper respiratory tract, but in the lungs at 37°C replication is inhibited. As a result, the virus has lost its virulence in the human host and does not cause clinical influenza. Because of the intrinsic unpredictability of the formation of natural reassortants, extensive safety research has been done to demonstrate that the *ca* viruses are genetically stable and do not convert back to the wild-type virus.[38] Based on these studies, the chances of a sudden emergence of a pathogenic influenza virus following the use of the live virus vaccine are considered remote.

Many placebo-controlled studies with LAIVs have been carried out, among children as well as adults.[38–40] These studies have shown that the LAIV is safe and efficacious. Some studies suggest that the LAIV might induce a certain degree of cross-protection against drift viruses, possibly due to its ability to induce a CTL response.[40] Another potential advantage of the LAIV may be its potential ability to dampen the spread of virus in the community, particularly if the vaccine were to be used widely among children.[38] However, theoretically, the same would be true for conventional inactivated vaccines. Clearly, the potential advantages of LAIVs over inactivated vaccines need further scientific demonstration and confirmation.

In several clinical trials, intranasal LAIV has been compared directly with conventional intramuscularly administered inactivated vaccines. A meta-analysis of these vaccine-controlled clinical trials has shown that mucosal sIgA antibody titres were higher after vaccination with LAIV, while inactivated vaccines induced higher serum IgG antibody titres.[41] In studies where culture-positive influenza illness was assessed, both vaccine types were found to be equally effective.

In the first year of FluMist® being on the market in the USA, a limited number of doses were sold, in part due to its extraordinarily high price and strict cold-chain distribution requirements. In addition, concerns remain about the use of live-virus vaccines in immunocompromised patients; indeed, health care workers vaccinated with LAIV have been advised not to be in contact with such patients for up to 3 weeks.[42] Clearly, more experience with this vaccine is required to relax the safety concerns that some people have. If the theoretical advantages of the LAIV can be scientifically substantiated and the safety concerns about the use of LAIV prove unwarranted,[38] FluMist® may well offer interesting new possibilities to control annual influenza epidemics.

In addition to the cold-adapted virus vaccines, novel recombinant influenza viruses, designed by modern reverse genetics techniques (see below), have been advocated as potential LAIVs. These include viruses with deletions in the NS1, enhancing their interferon sensitivity,[5] replication-incompetent NS2 knockouts[43] or viruses with attenuating mutations in M2.[44]

Novel approaches to vaccine virus production

While a number of experimental influenza vaccines are based on the use of antigen produced by recombinant DNA technology or even rely of the use of DNA itself as immunogen, it is expected that in years to come the primary basis for influenza vaccine production will remain the initial production of the influenza virus. Novel developments in this respect relate to the possibility of generating seed viruses by modern reverse genetics technology, and the use of mammalian cell-culture substrates for virus growth.

Reverse genetics

Reverse genetics provides a powerful technology for generation of recombinant influenza viruses with a desired combination of genes.[2] Previously, exchange of gene segments between different influenza viruses relied on deliberate reassortment, through co-infection of cells with two different viruses (see pp. 45–67). In this manner, high-growth reassortants have been generated for decades, to provide seed viruses for production of vaccine virus in chicken embryos.

Until recently, negative-strand viruses, such as influenza, have been refractory to reverse genetics approaches. The reason is that the viral genome consists of negative-sense RNA segments with unmodified 5' and 3' ends, which are replicated by a complex polymerase. Early reverse-genetics systems employed in vitro transcription of negative-sense RNA, transfection of this RNA along with purified polymerase proteins, and rescue of the transfected gene segment with a helper virus.[2]

More recently, cDNA vectors have been designed which allow transcription of the negative-sense viral RNA (using RNA polymerase I promoters) and positive-sense mRNA (using RNA polymerase II promoters) within cells.[5,45] This allows efficient production of viruses entirely on the basis of the eight desired recombinant gene segments through transfection of the DNA vectors into cells (Figure 33).

Reverse genetics techniques provide great opportunities to rapidly produce seed viruses for vaccine virus production either in eggs or in cell-culture substrates (see below). Drawbacks include the biosafety restrictions that apply to the generation and production of these recombinant influenza viruses and the complex intellectual property situation around this technology, which both hamper its unrestricted application.

Cell-culture vaccines

Influenza virus can be propagated efficiently on a number of cell-culture substrates. Currently, three cell lines are being developed for the production of influenza vaccine virus.[46,47] Two of these, MDCK and Vero cells, are dog and monkey kidney cells respectively. The third, the Per.C6 cell line, originates from a human embryonic retina cell. Among these cell lines, Vero cells in particular have a long history in human vaccine production. For example, poliovirus vaccine is produced on Vero cells. Two inactivated cell-culture influenza

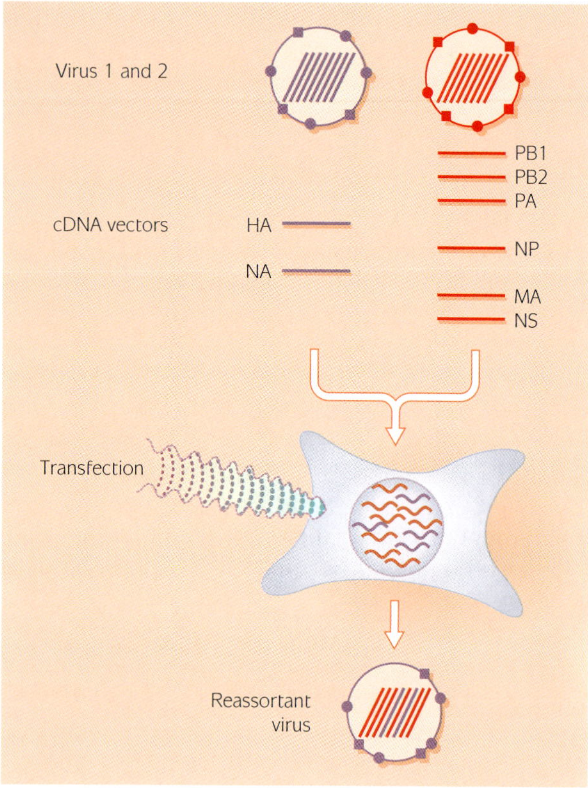

Figure 33. Schematic representation of the reverse-genetics technique for production of recombinant influenza viruses. A set of eight bidirectional transcription plasmids encoding the desired combination of influenza virus gene segments is transfected into cells, for example by electroporation. These plasmids produce messenger and as well as viral RNAs, ultimately resulting in the formation of new virus particles. Figure courtesy of Ron Fouchier, ErasmusMC, Rotterdam, The Netherlands.

vaccines, one produced on MDCK cells, the other on Vero cells, have already been licenced in Switzerland and the Netherlands, the latter as a Reference Member State (RMS) within the context of the Mutual Recognition Procedure (MRP) for the licensing of vaccines within Europe.

Extensive clinical evaluation of an inactivated influenza subunit vaccine, produced from virus grown on MDCK cells, has shown that it is safe and as immunogenic as subunit vaccine produced in eggs.[48,49] Also, MDCK- and egg-derived vaccines show comparable reactogenicity.[48,49] Likewise, Vero-produced whole virus vaccine appears safe and immunogenic. Growth of vaccine virus in cell-culture substrates is also economically feasible – indeed, a number of recent A strains of influenza, as well as the prototype A/PR8 virus, have been produced on an industrial scale.

Clearly, cell-culture-based vaccine virus production provides a great deal of flexibility. Virus production may be scaled up at short notice, such that unanticipated vaccine demands can be met. This is of particular importance in the case of pandemic threat. Accordingly, the WHO has recognized the need for development of cell-culture techniques for the production of influenza vaccines, supplemental to or as an alternative for egg-based vaccine production.[50] In addition, efficient propagation of virus on cultured cells does not require the generation of high-growth reassortants. This is another important time-saving advantage of cell-culture-based vaccine production. Furthermore, virus produced on mammalian cells retains the antigenic characteristics of the original virus isolates, whereas during virus propagation in eggs variants with an altered antigenicity may be selected for. Finally, growth of vaccine virus in cell culture excludes the presence of contaminants that may be present in egg-grown vaccines, notably ovalbumin or other egg proteins causing occasional allergic reactions, or bacterial endotoxin derived from infected eggs.

Other ways of producing vaccine antigen

Influenza subunit vaccine can also be prepared without the prior growth of the entire influenza virus. Rather, HA and/or NA may be produced in insect cells using a baculovirus expression vector. An experimental recombinant HA subunit vaccine produced in this manner,

FluBlØk™, has been evaluated in Phase I clinical trials with promising results.[51]

How may influenza control be further improved?

Improvement of vaccine use in target groups

Despite the well-established efficacy and effectiveness of current inactivated influenza vaccines, vaccination rates among target populations are less than optimal. Clearly, the available vaccines are underutilized. For example, in the USA, only 31% of adults between the ages of 18 and 64 years who are at risk for serious complications due to influenza are being vaccinated at this point.[52] In spite of an overall decline in rates of hospitalizations and implementation of influenza vaccination programmes, hospitalization for acute lower respiratory tract infections has increased.[53] Future efforts in the area of influenza vaccine development need to focus on older adult and high-risk populations who stand to derive great benefit from more robust immunological responses to influenza.

Suboptimal use of influenza vaccines is often an issue of perception based on lack of proper information. All too often influenza is viewed as a comparatively mild disease that does not pose serious threats. Conversely, influenza vaccination is frequently considered as ineffective or even causing the flu. In addition, the current mode of influenza vaccine administration by injection represents a barrier for individuals with fear of needles.

Clearly, the single most important factor influencing the use of influenza vaccine is whether it is recommended by the doctor. Therefore, primary-care physicians have a major role to play in implementing influenza vaccination programmes. Table 21 lists a number of recommendations in this respect.

Towards universal flu vaccination

Influenza is a major cause of illness and suffering, not only for the elderly and people with underlying medical conditions, but also for children and healthy younger adults.

Possible actions by primary care physicians to stimulate vaccine uptake in target populations
• Mark and update the records of people recommended for vaccination.
• Send invitation letters together with information leaflets to people recommended for vaccination.
• Organize vaccination clinics to administer vaccine to as many target subjects as possible in a time-efficient way.
• Promote vaccination of family members of at-risk patients and health care personnel.
• Display appropriate informative material in the doctor's office.

Table 21. Possible actions by primary care physicians to stimulate vaccine uptake in target populations. Courtesy of Ted van Essen on behalf of the Dutch College of General Practitioners.

Even though in most countries children are not included in the target groups, they are increasingly under consideration for routine flu vaccination. It is generally accepted that children play an important role in the spread of influenza infections in communities. In addition, influenza among children is a significant cause of parental work loss. Furthermore, very small children may well be at increased risk for serious influenza-associated complications. For this reason the Advisory Committee on Immunization Practices (ACIP) in the USA has encouraged the routine vaccination of children aged 6–23 months.[54] While younger adults are generally not at risk for serious complications due to influenza, flu remains an important cause of work absenteeism, diminished work productivity and malaise interfering with off-work activities. This is why vaccination of working adults against influenza will become an increasingly important issue in the near future.

References

1. Nicholson KL, Wood JM, Zambon M. Influenza. *Lancet* 2003; **362**: 1733–1745.

2. Bilsel P, Kawaoka Y. New approaches to vaccination. In: Nicholson KG, Webster RG, Hay AJ, editors. *Textbook of Influenza*. Blackwell Science, 1998; pp. 422–434.

3. Kemble G, Greenberg H. Novel generations of influenza vaccines. *Vaccine* 2003; **21**: 1789–1795.

4. Rimmelzwaan GF, Osterhaus ADME. Influenza vaccines: new developments. *Curr Opin Pharmacol* 2001; **1**: 491–496.

5. Palese P, Garcia Sastre A. Influenza vaccines: present and future. *J Clin Invest* 2002; **110**: 9–13.

6. Beyer WEP, Palache AM, Baljet M, Masurel N. Antibody induction by influenza vaccines in the elderly: a review of the literature. *Vaccine* 1989; **7**: 385–394.

7. Provinciali M, Di Stefano G, Muzzioli M *et al*. Impaired antibody response to influenza vaccine in institutionalized elderly. *Ann NY Acad Sci* 1994; **717**: 307–314.

8. Webster RG. Immunity to influenza in the elderly. *Vaccine* 2000; **18**: 1686–1689.

9. Boon AC, Fringuelli E, Graus YM *et al*. Influenza A virus specific T cell immunity in humans during aging. *Virology* 2002; **299**: 100–108.

10. Nichol KL. The efficacy, effectiveness and cost-effectiveness of inactivated influenza vaccines. *Vaccine* 2003; **21**: 1769–1775.

11. Stephenson I, Nicholson KG, Wood JM, Zambon MC, Katz JM. Confronting the avian influenza threat: vaccine development for a potential pandemic. *Lancet Infect Dis* 2004; **4**: 499–509.

12. Podda A. The adjuvanted influenza vaccines with novel adjuvants: experience with the MF59-adjuvanted vaccine. *Vaccine* 2001; **19**: 2673–2680.

13. Snider DP. The mucosal adjuvants activities of ADP-ribosylating bacterial enterotoxins. *Crit Rev Immunol* 1995; **15**: 317–348.

14. De Haan L, Verweij WR, Holtrop M *et al.* Nasal or intramuscular immunization of mice with influenza subunit antigen and the B subunit of *Escherichia coli* heat-labile toxin induces IgA- or IgG-mediated protective mucosal immunity. *Vaccine* 2001; **19**: 2898–2907.

15. Babai I, Barenholz Y, Zakay-Rones Z *et al.* A novel liposomal influenza vaccine (INFLUSOME-VAC) containing hemagglutinin–neuraminidase and IL-2 or GM-CSF induces protective anti-neuraminidase antibodies cross-reacting with a wide spectrum of influenza A viral strains. *Vaccine* 2001; **20**: 505–515.

16. Ben-Yehuda A, Joseph A, Barenholz Y *et al.* Immunogenicity and safety of a novel IL-2-supplemented liposomal influenza vaccine (INFLUSOME-VAC) in nursing-home residents. *Vaccine* 2003; **21**: 3169–3178.

17. Hehme N, Engelmann H, Kuenzel W, Neumeier E, Saenger R. Immunogenicity of a monovalent, aluminum-adjuvanted influenza whole virus vaccine for pandemic use. *Virus Res* 2004; **103**: 163–171.

18. Stegmann T, Morselt HW, Booy FP, Van Breemen JF, Scherphof G, Wilschut J. Functional reconstitution of influenza virus envelopes. *EMBO J* 1987; **6**: 2651–2659.

19. Bron R, Ortiz A, Dijkstra J, Stegmann T, Wilschut J. Preparation, properties, and applications of reconstituted influenza virus envelopes (virosomes). *Meth Enzymol* 1993; **220**: 313–331.

20. Bungener L, Serre K, Bijl L *et al.* Virosome-mediated delivery of protein antigens to dendritic cells. *Vaccine* 2002; **20**: 2287–2295.

21. Huckriede A, Bungener L, ter Veer W *et al.* Influenza virosomes: combining optimal presentation of haemagglutinin with immunopotentiating activity. *Vaccine* 2003; **21**: 925–931.

22. Glück R, Moser C, Metcalfe IC. Influenza virosomes as an efficient system for adjuvanted vaccine delivery. *Expert Opin Biol Ther* 2004; **4**: 1139–1145.

23. De Bruijn IA, Nauta J, Gerez L, Palache AM. Virosomal influenza vaccine: a safe and effective influenza vaccine with high efficacy in elderly and subjects with low pre-vaccination antibody titers. *Virus Res* 2004; **103**: 139–145.

24. Morein B, Sundquist B, Hoglund S, Dalsgaard K, Osterhaus A. ISCOM, a novel structure for antigenic presentation of membrane proteins from enveloped viruses. *Nature* 1984; **308**: 457–460.

25. Rimmelzwaan GF, Baars M, Van Amerongen G, Van Beek R, Osterhaus ADME. A single dose of an ISCOM influenza vaccine induces long-lasting protective immunity against homologous challenge infection but fails to protect Cynomolgus macaques against distant drift variants of influenza A (H3N2) viruses. *Vaccine* 2001; **20**: 158–163.

26. Voeten JT, Rimmelzwaan GF, Nieuwkoop NJ, Lovgren-Bengtsson K, Osterhaus AD. Introduction of the hemagglutinin transmembrane region in the influenza virus matrix protein facilitates its incorporation into ISCOM and activation of specific CD8(+) cytotoxic T lymphocytes. *Vaccine* 2000; **19**: 514–522.

27. Rimmelzwaan GF, Nieuwkoop N, Brandenburg A *et al.* A randomized, double blind study in young healthy adults comparing cell-mediated and humoral immune responses induced by influenza ISCOM vaccines and conventional vaccines. *Vaccine* 2000; **19**: 1180–1187.

28. Webster RG. DNA vaccination: a potential future strategy. In: Nicholson KG, Webster RG, Hay AJ, editors. *Textbook of Influenza*. Blackwell Science, 1998; pp. 410–421.

29. Ulmer JB. Influenza DNA vaccines. *Vaccine* 2002; **20** (Suppl 2): S74–S76.

30. Neirynck S, Deroo T, Saelens X, Vanlandschoot P, Jou WM, Fiers W. A universal influenza A vaccine based on the extracellular domain of the M2 protein. *Nat Med* 1999; **5**: 1157–1163.

31. Heinen PP, Rijsewijk FA, de Boer-Luijtze EA, Bianchi AT. Vaccination of pigs with a DNA construct expressing an influenza virus M2-nucleoprotein fusion protein exacerbates disease after challenge with influenza A virus. *J Gen Virol* 2002; **83**: 1851–1859.

32. Waldman RH, Bond JO, Levitt LP *et al*. An evaluation of influenza immunization: influence of route of administration and vaccine strain. *Bull World Health Org* 1969; **41**: 543–548.

33. Boyce TG, Hsu HH, Sannella EC *et al*. Safety and immunogenicity of adjuvanted and unadjuvanted subunit influenza vaccines administered intranasally to healthy adults. *Vaccine* 2000; **19**: 217–226.

34. Plante M, Jones T, Allard F *et al*. Nasal immunization with subunit proteosome influenza vaccines induces serum HAI, mucosal IgA and protection against influenza challenge. *Vaccine* 2001; **20**: 218–225.

35. Mutsch M, Zhou W, Rhodes P *et al*. Use of the inactivated intranasal influenza vaccine and the risk of Bell's palsy in Switzerland. *New Engl J Med.* 2004; **350**: 896–903.

36. Ghendon Y. Cold-adapted, live influenza vaccines developed in Russia. In: Nicholson KG, Webster RG, Hay AJ, editors. *Textbook of Influenza*. Blackwell Science, 1998; pp. 391–399.

37. Maassab HF. Adaptation and growth characteristics of influenza virus at 25°C. *Nature* 1968; **213**: 612–614.

38. Glezen WP. Cold-adapted, live attenuated influenza vaccine. *Expert Rev Vaccines* 2004; **3**: 131–139.

39. Mendelman PM, Cordova J, Cho I. Safety, efficacy and effectiveness of the influenza virus vaccine, trivalent, types A and B, live, cold-adapted (CAIV-T) in healthy children and healthy adults. *Vaccine* 2001; **19**: 2221–2226.

40. Belshe RB. Current status of live attenuated influenza virus vaccine in the US. *Virus Res* 2004; **103:** 177–185.

41. Beyer WEP, Palache AM, De Jong JC, Osterhaus ADME. Cold-adapted live influenza vaccine versus inactivated vaccine: systemic vaccine reactions, local and systemic antibody response, and vaccine efficacy. A meta-analysis. *Vaccine* 2002; **20**: 1340–1353.

42. Centers for Disease Control and Prevention. Prevention and control of influenza. *Recommendations of the Advisory Committee on Immunization Practices (ACIP)* 2004; MMWR 28(RR-6).

43. Watanabe T, Watanabe S, Neumann G, Kida H, Kawaoka

Y. Immunogenicity and protective efficacy of replication-incompetent influenza virus-like particles. *J Virol* 2002; **76**: 767–773.

44. Watanabe T, Watanabe S, Kida H, Kawaoka Y. Influenza A virus with defective M2 ion channel activity as a live vaccine. *Virology* 2002; **299**: 266–270.

45. De Wit E, Spronken MI, Bestebroer TM, Rimmelzwaan GF, Osterhaus ADME, Fouchier RAM. Efficient generation and growth of influenza virus A/PR/8/34 from eight cDNA fragments. *Virus Res* 2004; **103**: 155–161.

46. Brands R, Visser J, Medema J, Palache AM, Van Scharrenburg GJ. InfluvacTC: a safe Madin Darby Canine Kidney (MDCK) cell culture-based influenza vaccine. *Dev Biol Stand* 1999; **98**: 93–100.

47. Kistner O, Barrett PN, Mundt W, Reiter M, Schober-Bendixen S, Dorner F. Development of a mammalian cell (Vero) derived candidate influenza virus vaccine. *Vaccine* 1998; **16**: 960–968.

48. Palache AM, Scheepers HS, De Regt V *et al*. Safety, reactogenicity and immunogenicity of Madin Darby Canine Kidney cell-derived inactivated influenza subunit vaccine. A meta-analysis of clinical studies. *Dev Biol Stand* 1999; **98**: 115–125.

49. Halperin SA, Smith B, Mabrouk T *et al*. Safety and immunogenicity of a trivalent, inactivated, mammalian cell culture-derived influenza vaccine in healthy adults, seniors, and children. *Vaccine* 2002; **20**: 1240–1247.

50. World Health Organization. Cell culture as a substrate for the production of influenza vaccines: Memorandum from WHO meeting. *Bull World Health Org* 1995; **73**: 431–435.

51. Lakey DL, Treanor JJ, Betts RF *et al*. Recombinant baculovirus influenza A hemagglutinin vaccines are well tolerated and immunogenic in healthy adults. *J Infect Dis* 1996; **174**: 838–841.

52. Glezen WP, Greenberg SB, Atmar RL *et al*. Impact of

respiratory virus infections on persons with chronic underlying conditions. *J Am Med Assoc* 2000; **283**: 499–505.

53. Nichol KL, Margolis KL, Wouremna J, von Sternberg T. Effectiveness of influenza vaccine in the elderly. *Gerontology* 1996; **42**: 274–279.

54. Centers for Disease Control and Prevention. Prevention and control of influenza. Recommendations of the Advisory Committee on Immunization Practices (ACIP). *MMWR* 2002; **51**(RR-3).

Appendix 1 – Useful Websites

For patients

US Centers for Disease Control – www.cdc.gov/flu

World Health Organization – www.who.int/mediacentre/factsheets/fs211/en/

US National Institute of Health – www.niaid.nih.gov/factsheets/flu.htm

US NIH Q&A – www.nlm.nih.gov/medlineplus/tutorials/influenza/id439101.html

European Influenza Surveillance Scheme – www.eiss.org/html/faq_influenza.html

EU Influenza Media Backgrounder – http://europa.eu.int/comm/health/ph_threats/com/Influenza/contribution01_en.pdf

European Vaccine Manufacturers – www.evm-vaccines.org/Influenzaanglais.htm

For health care professionals

US Centers for Disease Control – www.cdc.gov/flu

World Health Organization – www.who.int/csr/disease/influenza/en/

European Influenza Surveillance Scheme – www.eiss.org

European Agency for the Evaluation of Medicinal Products – www.emea.eu.int/

European Scientific Working Group on Influenza – www.eswi.org

EU Influenza Media Backgrounder – http://europa.eu.int/comm/health/ph_threats/com/Influenza/contribution01_en.pdf

European Vaccine Manufacturers – www.evm-vaccines.org/influenza.htm

Pandemic Influenza Planning in Canada – www.hc-sc.gc.ca/english/diseases/flu/pandemic.html

Appendix 2 – WHO Guidelines

Global Agenda for Influenza Surveillance and Control

These extracts have been taken from the WHO guidelines that can be found at:

- www.who.int/csr/disease/influenza/globalagenda/en/
- www.who.int/csr/disease/influenza/csrinfluenzaglobalagenda/en/

Objectives of the Global Agenda

- Provide impartial and prioritized guidance to all parties on research and development and national/global action for influenza control
- Support co-ordination of action for influenza control and surveillance
- Support implementation of identified priorities
- Support advocacy and fund raising

The Global Agenda has been developed for all those involved in activities to:

- Reduce morbidity and mortality from annual influenza epidemics
- Prepare for the next influenza pandemic
- Co-ordinate national and international action in influenza surveillance and control
- Advocate and raise funds

Major Themes in the Global Agenda

1. Improvement in the quality and coverage of virological and epidemiological influenza surveillance
2. Improvement in the understanding of health and economic burden of influenza, including benefits from epidemic control and pandemic preparedness
3. Expansion in the use of existing vaccines, particularly in developing countries and in high-risk groups and acceleration in the introduction of new vaccines

4. Increase in national and global epidemic and pandemic preparedness, including vaccine and pharmaceutical supplies

Priority activities and key actions to reduce morbidity and mortality from annual influenza epidemics and to prepare for the next pandemic

A. Strengthen disease and virological surveillance nationally and internationally

i. Enhance and integrate virological and disease surveillance
ii. Expand virological and disease surveillance
iii. Expand animal influenza surveillance and integrate with human influenza surveillance
iv. Improve data management, utilization and exchange

B. Increase knowledge on the health and economic burden of influenza

i. Strengthen the capacity in epidemiological and statistical techniques for studies on influenza disease burden
ii. Evaluate the clinical and economic burden of disease in countries where there is no recognition of influenza or no control policies are in place
iii. Re-evaluate the clinical and economic burden of influenza in countries where influenza control policies are in place

C. Increase influenza vaccine usage

i. Encourage assessment of disease burden and cost-effectiveness analyses
ii. Encourage countries to establish national policies and set immunization targets

iii. Promote awareness among policy makers, health care providers, and the public
iv. Encourage countries to identify and develop effective strategies for vaccine delivery
v. Develop and implement methods for the measurement and feedback of the progress of national and local programmes

D. Accelerate national and international action on pandemic preparedness

i. Increase awareness of the need for pandemic planning
ii. Accelerate the development and implementation of national pandemic plans
iii. Enhance the utilization of influenza vaccine and antivirals in the inter-pandemic period
iv. Develop strategies for the utilization of vaccines and antivirals and secure adequate supplies for a pandemic
v. Advocate research on pandemic viruses, vaccines, antivirals and other control measures

The Global Agenda on Influenza Surveillance and Control was developed and agreed by consensus by the participants of the WHO Consultation on Global Priorities in Influenza, World Health Organization, Geneva, Switzerland, 6–7 May 2002.

Influenza vaccines

The following extracts have been taken from a WHO position paper.[1]

WHO position paper

The current position paper, which is mainly concerned with the inter-pandemic influenza situation, is an interim publication pending further policy development by the WHO Global Influenza Programme.

> Data on vaccination coverage show that even in industrialized countries, large proportions of the population at risk do not receive the influenza vaccine. WHO therefore encourages initiatives to raise awareness of influenza and influenza vaccination among health care workers and the public, and encourages setting of national targets for vaccination coverage.

The justification for vaccine use

During influenza epidemics, attack rates of 1–5% are most commonly observed, but the attack rate may reach 40–50% or more among elderly persons in institutions and in other high-risk groups. At least in western communities, bacterial complications such as pneumonia are frequently associated with influenza; the total annual excess mortality during influenza epidemics is estimated at 7.5–23 per 100,000. Influenza poses a considerable economic burden both on society and the individual in terms of consumption of health care resources and lost productivity.

Internationally licensed influenza vaccines have proven to be efficacious and safe. During influenza outbreaks, appropriate vaccination may significantly reduce respiratory illness and sick-leave among healthy adults. More importantly, vaccination may reduce severe disease and premature death in the elderly and in persons with underlying ailments or disease (for details on vaccine efficacy, see below).

Antiviral drugs such as the M2 inhibitors (acting against type A virus) and the more recently developed neuraminidase inhibitors (acting against both type A and type B viruses) have been shown to be effective for treatment (and for some agents, prophylaxis) and are now available in many industrialized countries. Resistant mutants to both classes of antiviral agents have been detected, and antimicrobial resistance surveillance is important to assess the magnitude of this problem. Also, costs, occasional side effects and the likely limited availability of such drugs during major outbreaks highlight the role of vaccination as the primary preventive measure against influenza.

Influenza virus vaccines

The three types of inactivated influenza vaccine show comparable efficacy, but differ in terms of reactogenicity. Thus in 15–20% of vaccines, the whole virus vaccines cause local reactions lasting for 1–2 days. Such reactions appear to be more common in young children than in adults. Transient systemic reactions such as fever, malaise and myalgias may occur in a minority of vaccine recipients within 6–12 hours of the vaccination. Split vaccines and subunit vaccines show reduced systemic reactogenicity both in children and in adults as compared to whole virus preparations. Consequently, subunit and split-virus vaccines are more attractive, particularly for use in children.

WHO position on influenza vaccines

The main purpose of influenza vaccination is to avoid severe influenza and its complications. This paper is concerned mainly with epidemic influenza and the public health impact of yearly influenza vaccination. Authoritative information on pandemics can be found in the WHO influenza pandemic plan. Recommendations for the use of inactivated influenza vaccines and other preventive measures are published in the weekly epidemiological record.

Most of the widely licensed influenza vaccines are manufactured according to the quality requirements defined by WHO and have proven efficacious in the elderly and other groups at risk. If influenza vaccination of children is required, for example as a consequence of predisposing conditions, the vaccine will not interfere with diphtheria–pertussis–tetanus (DTP) or other childhood vaccines, possibly due at the same time. To reduce adverse effects, only split vaccines or subunit vaccines should be given to children. Influenza vaccine should not be given to children aged under 6 months, and those aged 6–35 months should only receive half the adult vaccine dose.

Ideally, when major outbreaks are expected, all individuals should have the opportunity to be vaccinated against influenza. However, limited health budgets and, at least initially, shortage of the appropriate vaccine may force health authorities to restrict influenza vaccine to groups at particular risk. The following priority is recommended:

1. Residents of long-term care facilities for the elderly and the disabled – they are considered at high risk of influenza and its complications
2. Elderly non-institutionalized individuals suffering from chronic conditions such as pulmonary or cardiovascular illness, metabolic diseases including diabetes mellitus and renal dysfunction, and various types of immunosuppression including persons with AIDS and transplant recipients
3. All adults and children aged over 6 months suffering from any of the conditions mentioned above
4. Individuals who are above a nationally defined age limit irrespective of other risk factors. Although the appropriate age for general vaccination may be considerably lower in countries with poor living conditions, most countries define the limit age >65 years
5. Other groups defined on the basis of national data
6. Health care workers in regular, frequent contact with high-risk persons
7. Household contacts of high-risk persons.

Pregnant women who will be in their second or third trimester by the start of the influenza season and who are likely to be exposed are advised to consider vaccination in careful consultation with a competent healthcare provider. From a societal perspective, there are good arguments for influenza vaccination of children and healthy adults. Where adequate vaccine supplies are available, vaccination of the general public may be considered. However, the implementation of large-scale influenza vaccination programmes for these groups requires further evaluation of cost-effectiveness and cannot be generally recommended until firm data are presented. Nevertheless, persons who provide essential community services should be considered for vaccination. In some developed countries, companies find it economically justifiable to offer vaccination to their employees.

Although the WHO global influenza surveillance network has proven to be a reliable and successful system, it is important to increase worldwide coverage. Many countries are not included in the network, and in some large countries more than one centre is required. Surveillance is of particular importance in rural areas where potential animal hosts and humans live in close proximity, since it is in such areas that new viral recombinants are likely to originate.

[1] Influenza vaccines. *Weekly Epidemiological Record* 2002; **77**: 229–240.
http://www.who.int/docstore/wer/77_27_52.html

The relatively low uptake of influenza vaccines in most industrialized countries implies that significant proportions of the groups at risk of complications from influenza are not vaccinated. WHO strongly emphasizes the importance of raising the public consciousness of influenza and its complications as well as of the beneficial effects of influenza vaccination.

Appendix 3 – WHA Resolution

Fifty-sixth World Health Assembly WHA56.19

Agenda item 14.14 28 May 2003

Prevention and control of influenza pandemics and annual epidemics

- The Fifty-sixth World Health Assembly, Recalling resolutions WHA22.47 and WHA48.13;
- Recognizing that influenza viruses are responsible for seasonal epidemics that sicken millions worldwide and cause fatal complications in up to one million people each year;
- Further recognizing that many of these deaths could be prevented through increased use, particularly in people at high risk, of existing vaccines, which are safe and highly effective;
- Welcoming the contribution of global influenza surveillance, co-ordinated by WHO, to the annual determination of the antigenic composition of influenza vaccines and to early recognition of conditions conducive to a pandemic, and the assistance provided by WHO to timely manufacturing of influenza vaccines;
- Expressing concern that the health burden and economic impact of influenza in developing countries are poorly documented, and that recent evidence suggests higher rates of fatal complications associated with poor nutritional and health status and limited access to health services;
- Further concerned by the general lack of national and global preparedness for a future influenza pandemic, particularly in view of the recurrence of such pandemics and the high mortality, social disruption

and economic costs that they invariably cause and which may be exacerbated by rapid international travel, the recent worldwide increase in the size of at-risk populations and the development of resistance to first-line antiviral drugs;

- Recognizing the need for improved vaccine formulations, increased manufacturing capacity for vaccines, more equitable access to antiviral drugs, and strengthened disease surveillance as part of national and global pandemic preparedness;
- Noting that better use of vaccines for seasonal epidemics will help to ensure that manufacturing capacity meets demand in a future pandemic, and that pandemic preparedness plans will help to make the response to seasonal epidemics more rational and cost-effective as well as preventing numerous deaths;
- Noting with satisfaction the consensus reached by the WHO Consultation on Global Priorities in Influenza Surveillance and Control (Geneva, May 2002) on the first Global agenda on influenza surveillance and control, which provides a plan for co-ordinated activities to improve preparedness for both seasonal epidemics and a future pandemic;[1]
- Further noting with satisfaction WHO's work on influenza pandemic preparedness planning and its intention to draw up a model plan.

1. URGES Member States:

1. where national influenza vaccination policies exist, to establish and implement strategies to increase vaccination coverage of all people at high risk, including the elderly and persons with underlying diseases, with the goal of attaining vaccination coverage of the elderly population of at least 50% by 2006 and 75% by 2010;
2. where no national influenza vaccination policy exists, to assess the disease burden and economic impact of

annual influenza epidemics as a basis for framing and implementing influenza prevention policies within the context of other national health priorities;

3. to draw up and implement national plans for preparedness for influenza pandemics, giving particular attention to the need to ensure adequate supplies of vaccine, antiviral agents, and other vital medicines, as outlined in the Global Agenda on Influenza Surveillance and Control;
4. to contribute to heightened preparedness for epidemics and pandemics through strengthening of national surveillance and laboratory capacity and, where appropriate, increase support to national influenza centres;
5. to support research and development on improved influenza vaccines, and also effective antiviral preparations, particularly concerning their suitability for use in developing countries, in order to obtain an influenza vaccine formulation that confers long-lasting and broad protection against all influenza virus strains

2. REQUESTS the Director-General:

1. to continue to combat influenza by advocating new partnerships with organizations of the United Nations system, bilateral development agencies, nongovernmental organizations and the private sector;
2. to continue to provide leadership in co-ordinating the prioritized activities for epidemic and pandemic

preparedness set out in the Global Agenda on Influenza Surveillance and Control;

3. to provide support for developing countries in assessing the disease burden and economic impact of influenza and in framing and implementing appropriate national policies for influenza prevention;
4. to continue to strengthen global influenza surveillance as a crucial component of preparedness for seasonal epidemics and pandemics of influenza;
5. to provide technical support for Member States in the preparation of national pandemic preparedness plans, including guidance on estimating the demand for vaccines and antiviral drugs;
6. to search jointly with other international and national partners, including those in the private sector, for solutions to reduce the present global shortage of, and inequitable access to, influenza vaccines and antiviral drugs, and also to make them more affordable, both for epidemic and global pandemic situations;
7. to keep the Executive Board and Health Assembly informed of progress.

Tenth plenary meeting, 28 May 2003
A56/VR/10

[1]Global agenda on influenza – adopted version. Part I. *Weekly Epidemiological Record* 2002; **77**:179–182. Adoption of Global agenda on influenza – Part II. *Weekly Epidemiological Record* 2002; **77**: 191–195.
http://www.who.int/docstore/wer/77_1_26.html

Index

Notes

As influenza is the subject of this book, all index entries refer to influenza unless otherwise specified. Page numbers followed by 'f' indicate figures; page numbers followed by 't' indicate tables or boxed material.

A